Dr. Wilfrid E. Shute's
Complete Updated
VITAMIN E
BOOK

Dr. Wilfrid E. Shute's
Complete Updated
VITAMIN E
BOOK

Keats Publishing, Inc.   New Canaan, Connecticut

DR. WILFRID E. SHUTE'S COMPLETE UPDATED VITAMIN E BOOK

Copyright © 1975 by Wilfrid E. Shute

ISBN: 0-87983-088-3
Library of Congress Catalog Card Number: 75-7808

Printed in the United States of America

Keats Publishing, Inc.,
36 Grove Street, New Canaan, Connecticut 06840

CONTENTS

DEDICATION

THIS BOOK IS AFFECTIONATELY DEDICATED to my wife Dorothy, whose involvement in Vitamin E therapy is not less than my own. Through the years she has observed its effects at first hand. She has seen pitifully burned little bodies healed, has exulted with me over the salvage of diabetic legs and has rejoiced over the improvement of cardiac cripples and their return to normal living. In addition, she has played an active role of her own.

Besides sharing my joys and enthusiasms, my wife has taken an important, indeed essential, part in the development of the Shute Institute and in the enormous amount of secretarial work that has been required by the nature of my activities.

If it had not been for her efforts, the Shute Institute might well have died aborning. She willingly left our comfortable and happy home in Guelph, Ontario, to accompany me to

London, Ontario, where the Institute was about to open its doors. When we found nothing there but a desk, a chair, a lamp, a telephone and a wastebasket into which all inquiries, after being answered with a form letter, were dumped, she joined me in arranging for the furnishing of the Institute (which was accomplished in ten days) and in setting up appointments for my patients. Living in what had been servants' quarters of the home which now housed our clinic —the only ones available—and assisted only by a "nanny" brought from Guelph to look after our two little daughters, she took charge of the office, remaining until the Institute was a flourishing success. Fortunately for me, she is an expert stenographer, secretary and office manager.

When I decided to move to Port Credit, she again unhesitatingly moved with me to this suburb of Toronto—this in spite of a house she loved and a happy environment for herself and our two girls—one a fine student and figure skater, the other a fantastically successful swimmer. (Swimming, of course, was of great interest to my wife since she herself had represented Canada as a swimmer at the Olympics in 1928 and 1932.)

Since then, while caring for our children and our home unaided, she has taken care of my voluminous correspondence, often taking dictation in the early morning, at noon hour or late in the evening. She typed every word of the many articles I wrote for *The Summary*, a publication of the Shute Foundation, when in London, and every word of the manuscript of *Vitamin E for Ailing and Healthy Hearts*, which was published by Pyramid Books in 1969, and every word of the manuscript of this book as well. She has been a tower of strength, a wise critic and an understanding co-worker.

To my alter ego, then, Dorothy Prior Shute.

I should also like to express my appreciation for the continuous help and support of my nursing staff—the nurses at the Institute and those in my office in Port Credit—and especially Miss Ada Pascoe and Mrs. Ursulla Donaldson.

I must, of course, acknowledge the faith of my father and his inspiration, which was responsible for all three of his sons becoming doctors, and the unusual medical intuition and knowledge and truly scientific mind of my older brother Evan, who delivered my two girls and who involved me in the medical uses of Vitamin E.

FOREWORD

THIS BOOK somehow had to be written. Two circumstances, particularly, have made it mandatory. One is the crying need for a useful therapy to combat the rapidly growing epidemic of heart disease. The other is the obvious sterility of most current approaches to the problem. Together they have made it essential to alert physicians and the public to the fact that real help for heart disease is available through the use of alpha tocopherol (Vitamin E) in megavitamin dosages.

The success of my first book, *Vitamin E for Ailing and Healthy Hearts*, has convinced me that such books are a far more effective method of reaching people—both physicians and the general public—than are papers in medical journals. Laymen, of course, rarely read medical journals. Probably a great many doctors are too busy to do more than thumb through many of them unless they are looking for a particular

article. Most medical journals, moreover, are extremely con-
servative. Often they will condemn out of hand something
new when it first appears. Later, when evidence for its effectiveness mounts, they may be too embarrassed to print it.

My reasons for addressing physicians will be readily
apparent. Many doctors are now familiar with the role of
alpha tocopherol in the treatment of heart disease, arteriosclerosis, burns and other conditions. Many now use it in
their treatment of some of their patients. Many others, however, are not fully aware of the importance of this substance.
Many, in fact, are laboring under the misapprehension that
most of the claims for Vitamin E have not been substantiated.
For the sake of their patients and themselves, it is extremely
important that these physicians should become familiar not
only with the claims for this substance but with the extensive
and very solid evidence for them that is now available.

I address laymen as well because I know from experience
that those who come to understand the importance of what I
have to say can be enormously effective in spreading awareness of it. I am especially concerned that, as parents and
citizens, they should know the effects of some food processing techniques in removing important amounts of certain
essential constituents from some foods.

But there is still another reason for talking to laymen. I
hope that they will discuss this book with their doctors—if
necessary, making sure that these doctors see the book so that
they can evaluate it for themselves. Whether a physician
reads this book and alerts his patients, or whether a layman
reads it and alerts his physician, is all the same to me. What
matters is that people must know what alpha tocopherol can
do for them and for others before it is too late.

The immediate impetus behind the publication of this
book is the publicity given recently to some of the research on
the use of alpha tocopherol or mixed tocopherols in small

doses. Much of this material, in my opinion, has the potential for causing incalculable damage. Although the authors are usually capable of discussing the actions of small amounts (five to thirty international units [IU]) of alpha tocopherol, they generally have no experience with or knowledge of the uses of this substance at megavitamin levels (150 to 3,000 IU) in the treatment of human disease states. According to these writers, large quantities of Vitamin E are effective only in treating a few rare human abnormalities, a "rare form of anemia in premature infants" and intermittent claudication—leg pain that is due to severe arteriosclerotic narrowing of arteries in the legs.

Such articles are especially dangerous in that doctors have been influenced since grammar school days to consider their teachers as infallible. This attitude prevails even in medical school. Thus, they are likely to accept as gospel what they are told by professors of nutrition or biochemistry, even though the working lives of these people may be far removed from clinical medicine.

I have therefore gone to some length to report in their own words what doctors have said about what they can do *without Vitamin E therapy* in the treatment of cardiovascular disease and to contrast with this what other doctors have reported in medical journals that they can do *with Vitamin E therapy.* I leave it to the good judgment of the doctors who read this book whether, in all conscience, they continue using the old "crisis" approach to heart disease or save their patients by the intelligent application of new medical procedures including especially the use of alpha tocopherol.

I should like to add two final notes about this book and its organization in the hope that they will facilitate reading. The first concerns the method of presenting information. The second deals with the handling of references.

Since I have very consciously written this book both for

physicians and for laymen, I have tried to present information in a way that will be sufficiently clear for the latter and, at the same time, appropriate for the former. Wherever a brief explanatory paragraph or a few parenthetical definitions not needed by physicians may appear, I would hope that my physician readers will simply skip quickly ahead. I would hope, also, that this method will allow readers who are laymen to proceed easily and quickly with material that might otherwise have seemed overly technical.

Finally, in many publications, bibliographical references are grouped together in a special section at the back. This forces the serious reader to undertake the tedious and annoying task of turning continually away from the section he is reading to hunt for the supporting authorities elsewhere. In this book, such an arrangement has been avoided. Many of the publications mentioned in the text are referred to there in such a way that the reader will know instantly whose work is being discussed or quoted. Key sources are fully cited at the end of the chapters in which they are referred to. Additional references that I think may be useful appear at the end of Chapters 5 and 7.

WILFRID E. SHUTE, B.A., M.D.
Lake Worth, Florida.

1

THE HEART ATTACK AND YOU

SOME YEARS AGO a patient of mine who was recovering from a myocardial infarction (in laymen's language, a heart attack) remarked bitterly that he had led a clean life. This man was an athletic individual who had remained slim, who neither smoked nor drank and who got plenty of rest. Yet there he was, in the hospital, in spite of having avoided all the widely publicized pitfalls that are supposed to land you there. No question about it: he was angry.

I had to tell this man something that surprised him: that although the precautions he had taken were believed by many doctors to be valuable, they could not prevent a heart attack if a person's bloodstream contained an insufficient amount of one essential substance. Supplying this substance in adequate amounts would continue to be the most important part of his treatment. This substance, alpha tocopherol, constitutes the largest part, if not indeed the total amount, of the "antithrombin" (anti-clotting factor) in the human bloodstream.

The same statement applies to *you*, regardless of most of the efforts you may have made to stay healthy. Being slim and abstemious is fine. I certainly wouldn't deny that. But please put aside, for the moment, any idea that this gives you any reason to expect protection against a "heart attack," while you read some cold facts and figures.

The role of the antithrombin in such cases as this patient's will be elucidated in Chapter 3, and the relative unimportance of rest, exercise, and the avoidance of tobacco and alcohol will be stressed in the same chapter.

One difficulty in discussing the present epidemic of heart disease—and that is what today's situation is—is that nobody expects it to hit *him*. That seems to be the way our psychology works. Whether you, reading this book, are a doctor or a layman, you probably find it easier to imagine another person being vulnerable to a heart attack than to picture such a thing in relation to yourself. It's strange, when you think of it, that doctors are guilty of this kind of thinking, because this particular epidemic has hit the medical profession harder than most other groups!

Now I want you to pause for a few minutes to read some statistics and apply them consciously—first to *yourself*, then to *your family* and finally to *your friends*.

Statistics, I know, are dry. And huge figures, after a while, seem to convey very little meaning. We have all become so accustomed to reading about millions and billions today that the immensities they represent don't really sink in. For this reason I'll use percentages, rather than large numbers, as much as possible.

If you are a man over forty, your chances of dying of a myocardial infarction are better than 50 percent. Think about it. No matter how daring a gambler you are, this is frightening.

Statistics of the last twenty years suggest that although men predominate still, the rate of infarction in women is increasing steadily. And not all of these women are in the older age group. On 6 September 1971, the *Journal of the American Medical Association* contained a report concerning "myocardial infarction in two sisters less than 20 years old." The youngest proven infarction in a woman in my experience was in a twenty-five-year-old.

Equally startling—for I'm sure no one else has told you this—is the fact that this "disease" did not exist in 1900. Four cases of coronary thrombosis (heart attack resulting from obstruction of the coronary artery by a clot of blood) were the subject of an uncorroborated report in 1896 by Dr. George Dock (1). Coronary thrombosis remained almost entirely unknown, however, until it was described by Dr. J.B. Herrick (2) in 1912.

Most doctors are totally unaware of this. But it is a fact that has been specifically noted by Dr. Paul Dudley White, one of the two original cardiologists in America. Dr. White once wrote that at the time he graduated from medical school in 1911 *he had never heard of coronary thrombosis!* Sadly enough, Dr. White himself not long ago became the victim of repeated vascular episodes, the last of which was fatal.

I would say that your chances of dying of a myocardial infarction in 1912 were infinitesimal. Even in 1930, myocardial infarction was "an old man's disease." Yet today more than a million people each year in the United States die of cardiovascular diseases (diseases of the heart and blood vessels) and coronary thrombosis is the leading cause of these deaths.

Official statements concerning the magnitude of the epidemic are not hard to find. In 1968, the Inter-Society

Commission for Heart Disease Resources issued a startling report. The Commission stated that 600,000 persons die of heart disease each year in the United States. Of these about 27 percent are under sixty-five years of age. The Fall-Winter 1972 issue of the *American Heart*, a publication of the American Heart Association, placed the total number of Americans suffering from heart and blood vessel diseases at 27 million. About 80 percent of these are afflicted with hypertension, nearly 15 percent with coronary heart disease and nearly 6 percent with rheumatic heart disease. "Cardiovascular diseases," says the *American Heart*, "claim more American lives than all other causes of death combined." According to the same publication, heart attack claimed nearly 670,000 lives in 1969 and stroke—a common end result of hypertension (high blood pressure)—was responsible for about 207,000 more.

Comparable figures for heart attack deaths in Australia, Canada and Germany, are 60,000, 76,000 and 105,000 respectively. These deaths represent more than 50 percent of the total number of deaths in Austrialia and Canada and roughly the same percentage of the total deaths in Germany.

These, then, are the statistics. They probably won't have much impact unless you apply them to yourself and your family and until you think carefully about the fact that coronary thrombosis has not always been with us. In fact, it's a relatively recent phenomenon, as I have shown.

Another thought I want you to ponder long and well is that the medical profession has been unable to change this worsening picture. If there were a solution known to organized medicine, there would surely have been a significant drop in the death rate from coronary thrombosis, or at least a noticeable drop in its incidence, somewhere in the Western world. There has been, instead, a steady increase.

The third thought I want to plant firmly in your mind at

the outset is this. Up to the time this is being written, cardiologists have, for some strange reason, virtually always done everything wrong and never yet done anything right —an amazing situation which I shall explore in detail in a later chapter. Of course, I should add that there are quite a number of individual cardiologists who are now using what I know to be the correct method of preventing and treating coronary thrombosis. What I have said does apply, however, to cardiologists as a group—to the majority of people in the field.

If you become a heart patient, you will get no help from the usual cardiologist, except perhaps an accurate diagnosis. (You will also be treated for symptoms and complications, of course, but this does not really amount to getting assistance with your basic problems.) Nonetheless, you may well have to undergo dangerous and uncomfortable major procedures or take drugs which often cause side-effects and complications. And eventually your cardiologist may conclude that he cannot do much for you.

If a cardiologist believes that he cannot help you, he will sometimes refer you to a surgeon. In the surgeon's office you may be advised to undergo the latest in a rather long and growing list of surgical procedures, all except the current one having been used for periods ranging from months to years on thousands of patients by many enthusiastic, highly skilled surgeons. Yet each of these procedures has been abandoned in turn—which means that it proved useless, that the suffering and pain or death of the patients was in vain. At least, that is what I believe any thinking man or woman—and certainly any thinking doctor—must now conclude. And the current operation, in my opinion, may well be the worst of the lot.

The results of drug therapy have been similarly disappointing. Although some drugs give temporary relief, not one—with the exception of digitalis, which I shall discuss later—has been shown to improve the basic condition of the heart: they are effective only in removing symptoms, or in treating complications.

In the next chapter I shall demonstrate that drug therapy, surgery and another popular prescription—extended bed rest—are unlikely to solve the underlying problems of heart attack victims. Indeed, none of these will prevent a heart attack or (if you have been lucky enough to survive your first) will prevent further attacks.

I know that these are pretty sweeping statements. Whether you are a physician or a layman, I do not expect you to accept them without definite support from the medical literature and from statements by medical school professors and certified specialists in cardiology. These will be presented as I proceed.

I shall also substantiate what I say with a number of examples and case histories. (You will find many others—six or seven dozen, in fact—in my earlier book, *Vitamin E for Ailing and Healthy Hearts.*)

Some readers, I am sure, will already be convinced that what I am saying is true. They will have come to this conclusion because of their own experience or that of a family member or friend. If you are one of these, you may want to skip the next few chapters and go on to later sections of this book which will detail for you the very real help that has been available for the last twenty-seven years and that is now obtainable from a growing number of certified cardiologists and generalists in every civilized country in the world. For although the majority of doctors do not treat heart attack victims in the way I recommend, a great many now do.

If you are interested in the reasons why this different approach to cardiovascular disease is not more commonly used, you will find some of the later chapters of this book very enlightening. This is so, even though what these chapters contain amounts simply to a repetition of the experiences of very nearly every earlier pioneer in medicine—the experiences of Semmelweiss, Pasteur and Lister and, more recently, Banting and Best. The extremely important contributions of Dr. Carl J. Reich, Dr. Abraham Hoffer and Dr. Alan Cott, some of which I shall be discussing later, have also encountered the same kind of resistance.

Dr. Walter C. Alvarez (3) has summed up the situation very well. He states that in 1875, when Lister first spoke in the United States, physicians in the audience informed him that no surgeons in their home states used the method he had pioneered more than a decade before. And Alvarez recalls that in 1903 and 1906 Lister's work was still being ignored by some great American surgeons of Alvarez' acquaintance. It appears that the lessons of history must be relearned by each generation.

Please, reader, think carefully about what I shall tell you in this book. If you do not heed the information I shall give you, you have, as of now, no way of preventing a heart attack.

In October 1970, the *Medical Post* quoted Dr. Bernard Lown, Assistant Professor of Cardiology at Peter Bent Brigham Hospital in Boston, to the effect that 65 percent of those who sustain a "heart attack" in the United States die instantly or are dead on arrival at the hospital. Other sources have put the percentage considerably lower but still, think for a moment about Dr. Lown's statistic and what it means. Then think further about survival rates in the hospital. Depending on the statistics of different hospitals, your chance of dying if you reach the hospital alive may be as high as 40 percent, leaving you with a 21 percent chance of surviving the original attack. If you have already had a coronary thrombosis, you have no protection against another—and another is an altogether likely occurrence unless you do protect yourself, since you have already shown yourself to be susceptible to intravascular clotting (formation of blood clots in the vessels) which is the immediate cause of such attacks in most instances.

Believe me, I do not enjoy telling you this. I certainly don't want to alarm you unnecessarily, but I think it is better to know these things than not to know them. And I can offer you something positive: the information that there is a way to prevent heart attacks by providing the bloodstream with an adequate amount of a substance it requires which is known as alpha tocopherol or "Vitamin E." I shall tell you what it is, how and why it works in this way, and why many doctors today are using it more all the time, or are at least willing to try it.

So please, read on and consider what I have to say. I know you won't accept anything you read—whether it's by me or anyone else—without evidence. And of course you shouldn't. But do look at the evidence I shall present, and think about what it means.

You may live longer because you did.

REFERENCES

1. Dock, G. *Journal of the American Medical Association* 113, 563, 1939.
2. Herrick, J.B. *Journal of the American Medical Association* 59, 2015, 1912.
3. Alvarez, W.C. *Geriatrics* 25, 61, 1970.

2

WARNING: HOSPITAL AHEAD

DRUG THERAPY, BED REST AND SURGERY were mentioned in Chapter 1 as popular modes of treatment that are unlikely to solve the underlying problems of heart attack victims. I said that in general these methods don't work and that I would support this statement with references to medical literature and authorities. This means that this present chapter is going to be mainly negative in tone, but I don't see any way around that. After all, I can hardly expect any sensible person to accept new ideas unless I can first demonstrate that the old ones have to be replaced.

To help you to see what's wrong with the usual kind of treatment, let me start by asking you to imagine that you are a heart attack victim who has been lucky enough to reach the hospital alive. Let's assume that the doctor you get, on this occasion, is one who follows conventional procedures. Now let's see what happens.

21

There are several kinds of treatment that may be given to you, depending mostly on the tradition of the hospital you're in, the extent to which its practices are dominated by the views of the department heads—and what these views may be. Most or all of these will probably be familiar to you; they certainly will be, of course, if you are a doctor.

You may, for example, be placed in an intensive care unit or in a special version of this called a coronary care unit, and there hooked up to a monitor. You will be given morphine to decrease or remove the pain arising from the anoxic (oxygen-starved) heart muscle. (Besides morphine's pain-killing function, its second job, according to the textbooks, is to "allay apprehension.")

You may be kept in bed for six weeks or longer, with or without oxygen at the beginning of this period. In most hospitals the patient admitted following an acute coronary occlusion is put in an oxygen tent—which very likely has very little value, since the area of the heart causing the symptoms is the area deprived of blood supply by obstruction of the artery or arterial branch that had been supplying it—and oxygen, therefore, cannot get by the obstruction. Being put in an oxygen tent can distress the patient and is therefore useful chiefly in satisfying the relatives that something worthwhile is being done.

You may also be given oral or intravenous vasodilators, or both. These drugs tend to dilate the coronary artery, and some of them have a very brief action span. And you may be given anticoagulants (drugs which prolong the prothrombin time and so delay clotting in the blood).

I shall have quite a lot to say about anticoagulants. But before I go into this, let me make one thing clear. Even though I am skeptical concerning the value of drugs in general to alter the basic, underlying condition of the heart, it is our custom now, in treating cardiac patients, to use all useful and sensible forms of treatment available, even though all the drugs except digitalis are for symptomatic relief. (As to digitalis, I shall, as I have said, deal with this in some detail in later chapters.)

The one exception to this custom is anticoagulants. These we do not use.

The history of the widespread use of anticoagulant drugs, of which there are several, begins with the publication in 1948 of a paper by Drs. I.S. Wright, C.D. Marple and D.R. Beck (1). They stated that anticoagulants, given for the first four weeks after acute myocardial infarction, reduced the mortality rate by approximately one-half. This report was immediately confirmed by others and the treatment was very quickly adopted by virtually all cardiologists and soon afterward by nearly all general practitioners.

Following its introduction, many thousands of patients were subjected to this treatment. New laboratory facilities were set up and technicians were hired and trained to move around the wards taking blood samples, running prothrombin (clotting) times, entering figures on charts and keeping nurses and doctors busy adjusting patients' doses. In many cases, anticoagulant therapy was continued for months or years after the patient left the hospital. These drugs caught on to such an extent that at one time a physician could actually be accused of malpractice for not using them!

Yet in 1959, a report (2) concerning complications appeared in *The Lancet*. It said that among 217 patients treated with anticoagulants for up to three years, 105 had had a total of 194 bleeding episodes. Of these 139 were mild, 31 moderate and 24 severe. Three of the twenty-four died of hemorrhages. The scientist who analyzed the situation recommended that such treatment might best be restricted to "patients who can be expected to understand the dangers involved in this treatment and to recognize bleeding at the earliest possible moment."

In 1962 an editorial in the *Canadian Medical Association Journal* took note of reports which, it said, "cast doubt" on the value of anticoagulant therapy. "Among these, a retrospective survey and a large clinical trial in Copenhagen have tended to confirm the impression that mortality is practically identical in treated and control groups. . . . Apparently the mortality rate from myocardial infarction must be due mainly to causes that are unaffected by anticoagulants."

The same editorial went on to mention other reported complications: cardiac rupture, hemopericardium (blood collecting inside the sac which encloses the heart) and subdural hematoma (blood collecting under the outer lining of the brain inside the skull). The possibility that "minor degrees of intracranial bleeding are probably not uncommon as a complication of this form of treatment" was also mentioned. It was suggested that among patients with acute myocardial infarction, only those with complicating venous thrombosis and/or pulmonary embolism (blood clot or clots in the lung) might eventually be considered as having "the only certain indications for the administration of anticoagulants."

Since then, many more articles have appeared, such as that in 1962 by Dr. Richards (3) in the *British Medical Journal*. Richards found that mortality "remained constant, at about 33 percent whether or not patients were given anticoagulants." Drs. Liebow and Badger (4), writing in a 1963 issue of the *Journal of Chronic Diseases*, came to much the same conclusion. "The mortality rate in patients who did not receive anticoagulants," they said, "was similar to the rate in those who did."

In the following year an article by Drs. Brown and Mac-Millan in the *Canadian Medical Association Journal* stated that the use of heparin (an anticoagulant) in acute myocardial infarction and acute coronary insufficiency had been accepted without controlled clinical trial. Brown and MacMillan, in a study of their own, concluded that early intermittent intravenous heparin treatment did not cut mortality in patients with acute myocardial infarction. It also failed, they said, to "prevent impending myocardial infarction in patients with acute coronary insufficiency."

In 1965 the same authors discussed the literature on anticoagulants in the same journal. An abstract of that article summarizes it by saying that the authors' experience with them has been disappointing and that their review of the literature "has failed to establish benefit when all patients with coronary artery disease are treated with anticoagulant drugs." It was concluded that (after about eighteen years) there was a need for well-controlled studies of anticoagulant therapy.

In 1967, also in the *Canadian Medical Association Journal*, Dr. J.F. Mustard summed up the situation as to long-term therapy in the wake of myocardial infarcts in the following words: "Despite initial reports of a substantial benefit for treated patients, subsequent studies with adequately treated and control groups showed only a marginal benefit. There appears to be a moderate reduction in the frequency of new infarcts and some decrease in mortality." He noted that in most of the studies, the benefits were evident only in patients under sixty and that the benefits must, in any case, be "evaluated against the complications . . . in particular, hemorrhage."

At the thirty-ninth scientific session in 1967 of the American Heart Association, Dr. Arthur J. Seaman and colleagues at the University of Oregon reported the results of a ten-year double-blind study on the use of anticoagulants. These investigators recommended discontinuance of all long-term prophylactic (preventive) therapy with these drugs.

An editorial (5) in the *British Medical Journal* in 1970 reviewed the published reports and concluded: "The inherent danger of this form of treatment, together with the absence of any evidence of benefit, indicates that the time has come to abandon the long-term use of anticoagulants after myocardial infarction."

Perhaps the most complete recent summation is to be found in an editorial published in August 1970 in the *Journal of the American Medical Association* with the interesting title, "An Exercise in Futility." It refers to a report (6) from an international review group with members from Sweden, Canada (including Brown and MacMillan), Denmark, the United States and the United Kingdom who were unable to reach any definite conclusions but agreed on the need for future controlled trials of anticoagulant drugs.

The editorial asks: "Is there really a need for such trials? . . . Surely, years of experience with thousands of patients should have led by now to unequivocal conclusions, had anticoagulants in fact, played an important prophylactic role." It is concluded that additional studies might be "exercises in futility."

Think of the number of years it took university professors, cardiologists and others to discover this! And think of the fact that this form of treatment is still being used at this moment in most hospitals! Surely doctors who do this must know by now that its usefulness has been seriously questioned and that there are definite dangers. Nevertheless, this treatment continues to be used!

Such a situation highlights a major problem in science. This is that the opinion of the majority is very often wrong. One suggested new treatment may be adopted quickly and readily, yet another that is just as effective or more so may be ignored. Worthwhile advances in medicine are too often adopted slowly by the minority and in too many cases meet immediate, unreasoning opposition from politically prominent members of the medical profession and from doctors who are reluctant to admit that they don't know everything about everything. If a report casts doubt on an accepted practice, it can be a long time before its message is fully implemented.

At the beginning of this chapter I mentioned that if you were a heart attack patient you might be kept in bed for six weeks or longer. Strict bed rest for six weeks, followed by a six-week gradual return to activity, was the treatment universally used until about 1951, and it is still used in many places. Many hospitals, however, now stress early ambulation—a much better approach. They'll get you up after the first few days and send you home at the end of three weeks. But even in these hospitals, it's customary to immobilize a heart attack victim in the intensive care unit or coronary care unit for the first few days.

Hospitals are proud of their intensive care units with their expensive equipment, their specially trained nurses and the nearness of emergency resuscitation teams. You have probably developed a high regard for their efficiency. You may therefore be surprised to learn that although many cardiologists have reported decreased death rates in such units, others have questioned their value.

A report in a 1963 issue of *Applied Therapeutics* quotes a paper by Drs. Brown, MacMillan, Forbath and Mellagrani concerning such a unit in the Toronto General Hospital, a teaching hospital affiliated with the University of Toronto. The report states that an intensive care unit was set up "because of the distressingly high mortality (40 per cent) among patients with coronary thrombosis" in the hospital. Later that same year this same group (7) stated that the death rate had dropped *to 36 percent*, a statistically insignificant difference.

At the Rigshospital in Copenhagen, according to Professor Tybjaerg Hanse, the mortality rate among those admitted to the coronary care unit actually *rose* from 31.4 percent to 40.4 percent.

Some, though not all, other reports are more favorable. But except for one study which claims a reduction from 33 to 19 percent through the use of a coronary care unit, the papers I have seen generally suggest an immediate mortality rate of 36 to 40 percent.

In sharp contrast with these rates was the rate of 9.9 percent achieved in a study reported by Dr. S.A. Levine in the *American Heart Journal* in 1951 and in the *Journal of the American Medical Association* in 1952. (I have referred to Dr. Paul Dudley White as one of America's two original cardiologists. Dr. Levine is the other.) In these papers back in 1951 and 1952 Dr. Levine wrote that by merely sitting coronary thrombosis patients up in comfortable armchairs as soon as they were out of pain, and by giving them bathroom privileges, he had dropped the death rate to 9.9 percent.

Like many other great discoveries, this one was actually very simple! Dr Levine had difficulties, however, in gaining the cooperation of the patient's physician, the residents, interns and nurses. The very title he used to introduce his findings, "The Myth of Bed Rest in the Treatment of Coronary Thrombosis," suggests that he knew he was flying in the face of much well-established practice.

A Swedish study (8) reported in 1958 also achieved good results with this method. One group of 112 patients was treated in armchairs and given anticoagulants. Another one hundred patients were treated in armchairs but without anticoagulants. A third group of eighty was treated with bed rest and anticoagulants. The mortality rates were 10, 15 and 26 percent respectively. (About half of the subjects had had previous myocardial infarctions, whereas Dr. Levine's patients were a group in which about one-third had earlier coronary thrombosis in their histories.)

The *Journal of the American Medical Association*, summarizing the Swedish report in 1959, stated that the purpose of the armchair in that study "was not to increase the effort of the patients, but, on the contrary, to ease the burden of the heart muscle . . . Armchair treatment seemed to constitute a good prophylactic measure against embolic complications . . . . "*

The armchair treatment has been shown to be much superior to bed rest, and fortunately it is gaining headway in certain places—for example, in the Harper Hospital in Detroit. Other centers, rather than accept this radical change, have compromised on intensive care for the first few days with early ambulation and discharge within three weeks.

To the extent that early ambulation is now accepted as the correct treatment, the accepted treatment preceding it must have been wrong—not just not good, but very wrong. The statistics suggest, in fact, that it must have killed many coronary victims who would otherwise have survived.

Similarly, it is obvious that the coronary care unit today is more effective in reassuring the patient's family and friends than it is in treating the patient. It may well be that many of the arrhythmias (irregularities in a person's heartbeats) and cardiac arrests that are detected by their sophisticated equipment would not occur if only Dr. Levine's simple but radical procedure were followed.

You will have noticed, by now, that I am less than enthusiastic about anticoagulants and bed rest. I am equally

*In the same summary it was stated that although all three groups were more or less comparable in the severity of patients' infarctions, there was "a somewhat lower percentage of severe cardiac infarction in the armchair group receiving anticoagulants." It was also noted that most of the patients who died had developed arrhythmias or heart block (a problem that affects transmission of the heartbeat from the upper to the lower part of the heart). The summary concludes with the comment that it was probably "sufficient to treat only the bad prognostic risks (those with arrhythmias, heart block, and cardiac failure) with anticoagulants."

skeptical about the value of surgery for heart attack victims.

Great advances in the fields of anesthesia and surgical technique have made it inevitable that surgeons would become involved with the heart. And the development of mechanical pumps and artificial valves and of the ability to lower the patient's body temperature have made heart surgery progressively safer. Surgeons, accordingly, have devised many procedures for the correction of congenital anomalies, lesions caused by rheumatic fever, and coronary artery disease and its symptoms. They have had a distinct advantage in that they did not have the incubus of the double-blind study hanging around their necks. None of the surgical procedures has ever been subjected to close "scientific" scrutiny before being proposed, carried out, reported and generally adopted!

Certainly heart surgery which corrects congenital anomalies constitutes a great victory for medicine. The ablation of persistent ductus arteriosis, for example, leads to complete recovery. (This is a condition in which a blood vessel connecting the pulmonary artery to the aorta fails to close off, as it should, before a child is born. Ablation is the procedure for correcting this.)

Surgery for coronary artery disease, however, is something entirely different.

An editorial in the *Journal of the American Medical Association* for 27 July 1970 lists some of the procedures used during the preceding twenty-five years in surgery for coronary artery disease. Among them are:

- cervical ganglionectomy (removal of nerve cells near the upper end of the spinal cord in order to prevent certain impulses from reaching the heart muscle)

- thyroidectomy or radioactive iodine thyroid

ablation (two different methods of removing the thyroid gland in order to reduce metabolic demands on the heart muscle)

- various procedures such as epicardiectomy (surgical removal of part of the outer sac surrounding the heart) and omental grafts (a procedure involving a membrane in the abdominal area) for the purpose of inducing collateral circulation (making it possible for other blood vessels to do the work of vessels in the heart that have been damaged).

Although the editorial notes a revival of interest in myocardial revascularization (surgical grafting to reestablish blood supply to the heart muscle) and encouraging reports on results of surgery, it also presents results of a study comparing surgically treated patients unfavorably with a group of medically treated patients, in spite of the fact that the patients in the latter group were more seriously ill.

Although 14 percent of the medically treated group, as compared with only 9 percent of the surgically treated group (patients who had had double arterial implantation) had myocardial infarctions during the ensuing two-year period, only 9 percent of the medically treated patients died during that time, as compared with 30 percent of the surgical group. Moreover, signs of improvement (as measured by exercise tolerance and electrocardiograms) were present in 88 percent of the medical as compared with only 20 percent of the surgical patients. (Drs. Russek and Zohman, who treated the "medical" group, used propranolol [Inderal], a drug that slows down the heart and reduces its need for oxygen, and isosorbide dinitrate, a drug that dilates the blood vessels and increases blood flow to the heart muscles, plus prescribed exercise.)

It should be noted that each of the surgical procedures listed in this editorial was used on thousands of patients —and then abandoned for another procedure. Also, in contrast with the lengthy efforts involved before a new drug is approved, it would appear that new surgical procedures often are adopted with haste. This year's "new operation" may be next year's admitted failure. It is interesting also that the plethora of newspaper publicity that often accompanies surgical procedures—the naming of the surgeon, his picture in the paper, etc.—would lead to the expulsion of the purely medical man from his profession were he to court publicity in this manner.

Like the physician, however, the surgeon readily—and without apology—abandons a mistaken procedure. The heart transplant procedure is a case—though only one case—in point.

When it was announced amid world-wide fanfare that Dr. Christian Barnard had done the first transplant operation, many others rushed into the field, often without adequate preparation. The picture was really appalling. According to the *Medical Post* (6 May 1969), Dr. William R. Drucker, at that time Professor of Surgery at the University of Toronto and Surgeon-in-Chief of the Toronto General Hospital, told the annual conference of the Hospital Public Relations Officers Association of Australia that "many hospitals are carrying out heart transplants as publicity devices, without any intention of doing serious heart transplant research." Heart transplants, he said, were causing jealousy and rivalry between hospitals. Dr. Norman Shumway stated in a 1970 issue of *California Medicine* that some surgeons displayed "almost irresponsible haste to get in on the acclaim." He added that it was "almost a political thing."

According to his wife, the first recipient, Dr. Philip Blaiberg, afterward lived a life of agony. Of the 594 days he lived with a new heart, Blaiberg spent 248 in a Cape Town hospital fighting for his life. Of his days at home he spent ninety-five in bed.

The first transplant was done on 3 December 1967. By August 1970 only Dr. Shumway's surgical team was doing the operation and he was doing only ten a year. In all, 161 transplants were done, and nearly all the patients soon were dead. The cost of a single heart transplant was said to be 75 thousand dollars.

At the time of writing, the "latest operation" is the coronary artery bypass technique developed in 1967 by surgeons in Cleveland and Milwaukee. Where a patient's coronary artery has been narrowed by disease, a segment of the saphenous vein (a large vein in the leg) is connected to a diseased branch of the coronary artery above and below the narrowed area to serve as an alternate route for blood that would normally have passed through the coronary artery. The use of this technique has spread rapidly; it has been estimated that by early 1974 approximately a hundred thousand such operations had been performed. Opinion concerning the operation has not been unanimously favorable.

At the annual convention of the American Medical Association in 1971, a distinguished cardiologist, Dr. Eliot Corday, stated that although about twenty thousand of these revascularizations had been done within the preceding year, there was a lack of information about survival which made it hard to be certain about the kinds of cases in which the operation should be recommended.

Excerpts from Dr. Corday's remarks were published as an editorial in the *Journal of the American Medical Association* (9). "We already know," he says, "that one year after revascularization about 22 percent of vein grafts are occluded, 18 percent of patients have sustained a myocardial infarction, and cardiac function is worsened in 50 percent of those with previous myocardial damage." He goes on to note that "reliable statistics, which would enable us to determine if the new surgical procedures extend life, are not yet available for revascularization." Corday pleads for establishment of registries to study survival and results other than decrease in pain reported by angina patients. (Since patients with angina pectoris—a condition whose name means, literally, pain in the chest—have been known to gain relief from placebos and sham operations, such reports cannot be considered hard evidence by which to judge the success of revascularization.)

Later in 1972 Dr. David L. Brewer, Assistant Professor of Medicine at Duke University, reported that myocardial infarctions were common occurrences during coronary bypass surgery, with *one in five* patients undergoing the operation suffering a myocardial infarction on the table.

Also in 1972, doctors from the Montreal Heart Institute told the annual meeting of the Canadian Cardiovascular Society that following aorto-coronary surgery a high percentage of vessels become plugged up on the proximal side of the graft (the side closer to the origin of the vessel). A study had shown that occlusion occurred in 40 to 60 percent of coronary vessels not occluded (blocked) before surgery. Lack of clinical improvement, aggravation of symptoms and frequent occurrence of myocardial infarction following this operation are thus not difficult to understand!

It is interesting, in light of this, to note that on 22 February 1972 the *Medical Post* published an article in which it was suggested that reoperation was safe and effective for failing vein bypass grafts. The "latest thing" in 1967 was the bypass operation. In 1972 the "latest thing," presumably, was *reoperation* for failing bypass.

On 6 February 1974 a report appeared in my local newspaper in Florida, the *Palm Beach Post*, to the effect that Dr. John David Bristow of the University of Oregon was conducting a study designed to evaluate the coronary artery bypass. After nearly seven years and after a hundred thousand operations, a surgeon is trying to evaluate its effectiveness *on another sixty patients*!

On 4 March 1974 *Time* magazine carried a comment by Dr. Russek, now Professor of Cardiology at New York Medical College. Dr. Russek claimed, in the remarks quoted by *Time,* that drugs and other forms of medical care are far better treatment than surgery for most angina cases. He also stated that in his opinion more lives have been lost than saved through bypass surgery and that with "patients treated in one big city institution" there is a 66 percent probability of an unsuccessful result. Either they will suffer major complications or acquire a non-functioning graft or they will die on the table. He added that although deaths in the operating room may occur in fewer than 5 percent of cases, heart attacks, brain damage, hemorrhage, kidney failure or closure of the bypass were "not uncommon."

REFERENCES

1. Wright, I.S., Marple, C.D. and Beck, D.R. *American Heart Journal* 36, 801, 1948.
2. *The Lancet* 2, 489, 1959.
3. Richards, R.L. *British Medical Journal* 1, 820, 1962.
4. *Journal of Chronic Diseases* 16, 1013, 1963.
5. *British Medical Journal* 1, 514, 1970.
6. *The Lancet* 1, 203, 1970.
7. *The Lancet* 2, 349, 1963.
8. Helander, S. *Acta Medica Scandinavica* 162, 351, 1958.
9. Corday, E. *Journal of the American Medical Association* 219, 507, 1972.

3

A DIFFERENT APPROACH

"FOR THE PAST TEN TO FIFTEEN YEARS," says Dr. Eliot Corday, "a substantial number of patients have been following doctor's orders and avoiding risk factors. Yet the death rate from coronary artery disease is as high now as it was fifteen years ago."

Dr. Corday, a cardiologist at the University of California at Los Angeles, is also a member of the National Heart Advisory Council. The comment quoted above appeared in the *Los Angeles Times* of 2 April 1973. The "risk factors" mentioned in the article are commonly cited ones: "high cholesterol levels, smoking and sedentary habits."

The doctor's comments highlight a problem that bothers a lot of people who are concerned about their health.

From reading the last chapter, you will have gathered that treatment of people after they have had heart attacks leaves much to be desired. But what about the other obvious approach—prevention? Is the work being done there any better?

In the same interview, Corday summed up my own feelings about most of the research in the field of prevention. He said that as a researcher and a member of the Council he was familiar with the facts from the reports, and that these suggested to him that "we are on the wrong track." He suggested telling patients to avoid the so-called "risk factors" while warning them there is no real proof that this will work.

To think about prevention is always to think about causation. If a disease has been prevalent throughout medical history, this can be extremely difficult. But if a disease is relatively new, we have at least one good place to look for clues: the history of its emergence.

I have mentioned Dr. Paul Dudley White's statement that coronary thrombosis was unknown to him when he graduated from medical school in 1911. I have also given you the history of Dock's early report and Herrick's 1912 description. Further evidence that the present epidemic of cardiovascular disease is of quite recent origin is not hard to find. From 1926 to 1939, for example, deaths from coronary disease in Great Britain rose from forty-eight per million to 473 per million. In only thirteen years, a nearly tenfold increase!

The figures I have just quoted were mentioned in a 1946 address (1) by Sir Maurice Cassidy, who was Court Physician to King George VI. I refer to him not only because he happens to have set forth some startling information but because he went on to make a particularly acute observation. What he said was this: "The cause of coronary heart disease is still to seek . . . although an increasing number of investigators relate it to *nutritional deficiency of long duration*." (Italics mine.)

As I write today, Sir Maurice's comment is nearly thirty years old. I believed in the importance and value of the approach he mentioned at that time, and I believe in it now. I am convinced now, as then, that looking for causes is even more important than looking for cures, and that the basic and most important cause of cardiovascular disease is precisely a "nutritional deficiency of long duration." To explain why I think this, I shall first need to give those of you who are laymen a bit of background about the function of the heart and the proper role of clotting in the body.

The heart's function is to take blood which has just passed through tiny blood vessels in the lung, and thus been exposed to oxygen, and to push this oxygen-bearing fluid through other vessels to all the living cells in the body. The heart also takes blood returning from these cells through the veins and pushes it into and through the lungs. The left side of the heart does the former, the right side the latter. Blood, of course, contains many nutritive substances in addition to oxygen, and many other factors that maintain the health of the cells and protect them against damage.

The red cells in the blood, which actually carry the oxygen, pass through blood vessels which are, in many cases, very small. (In the smallest capillaries the cells must go through in single file.) Obviously there must be no clotting within the blood or the red cells will not be able to pass through the vessels. A clot anywhere within a blood vessel is therefore a catastrophe. Yet, under certain circumstances, blood must clot.

From time to time the body is subjected to various kinds of trauma (e.g., violent attack, accident, surgery) in which blood vessels are severed. When large vessels are involved, the blood flows out so rapidly that the victim will die very quickly unless proper first-aid measures are applied at once. More commonly, however, smaller vessels are involved, as in the case of the scratches, cuts and bruises we often see. If there were not a mechanism for the clotting of blood, the result would be fatal even in these minor cases. Therefore, the blood must contain substances which can form a clot which will occlude the cut ends of vessels, the surgically tied-off ends of severed vessels or the ruptured vessels involved in bruising.

Fundamentally, then, the problem is this. Except for the response of clotting when blood vessels are ruptured or severed, the blood must always remain fluid. When clotting is necessary, this must be confined to the area involved. And coronary thrombosis can only be avoided when the blood in the coronary arteries remains fluid.

Since coronary thrombosis was almost unknown before 1912, blood obviously did remain fluid up to that time. Only when it was needed to stop blood flow from a wound did the clotting factor spring into action. To me, the fundamental problem in all cardiovascular research is this: *What has happened, since 1912, to change this?*

It is obvious that the cause of coronary thrombosis, a condition which is unique to the last sixty years or so, must be connected in some way with the clotting mechanism in the bloodstream. Either something must have been added to the bloodstream that has made a difference, or something must have been taken away.

A number of environmental factors have been suspected, and some of these certainly may be involved to some degree. There are likely multiple factors in the increasing incidence of coronary thrombosis and myocardial infarction. It has been shown, for instance, that the hardness or softness of water may be a factor. Almost certainly the great increase in the use of refined starches, particularly white sugar, is a factor. A good case has been made for chlorination of drinking water as another. Certainly the use of literally thousands of additives in the processing of food, the great increase in pollution of air with heavy metals and the decrease in available clean water are possible contributors. *While possibly contributing, none of these factors can be of primary interest. Rather, the most likely basic explanation for the epidemic of heart disease we now have is the removal of some substance or substances from the environment and so from the bloodstream, substances essentially involved in the clotting mechanism.*

Obviously, before the epidemic, there must have been something in the bloodstream which controlled the clotting mechanism so that this essential process did not get out of hand, so that it was confined to the places and times where it was useful, indeed essential to life. As well as substances which activate and facilitate the clotting process, there had to be a chemical entity in the bloodstream to hold these in check. Long ago, scientists named this the *antithrombin* or anti-clotting factor.

Today, we know that the natural antithrombin in the bloodstream is a chemical called *alpha tocopherol*. Although this knowledge has been applied by only a relatively few members of the medical profession, it has been available for many years.

What kind of a chemical is alpha tocopherol?

Alpha tocopherol is one of a considerable number of organic compounds called vitamins which are needed if we are to live healthy lives and which, fortunately, can be found in foods. Alpha tocopherol is one of a group of compounds —the others being beta, gamma, delta, epsilon, eta and zeta tocopherol—which collectively are known as Vitamin E. It is an oil-soluble vitamin which is stored in fatty tissues of the body.

It was shown more than twenty years ago that a female body stores three times as much Vitamin E as a male body of like age and development. For many years this was apparently sufficient to give women greater protection against coronary heart disease. Unfortunately, this is no longer as true as it was, for reasons that I shall shortly explain.

Some of you, of course, will be familiar with the history of vitamins. For those who are not, let me provide a few necessary items of information.

Vitamins are a group of compounds whose existence and importance began to be uncovered early in the twentieth century. What has been called the "vitamin hypothesis" was set forth in 1911 by Casimir Funk, a Polish-born biochemist. It has been clearly established that there are certain vitamin deficiency diseases: scurvy, beriberi and rickets, for example. Vitamins in tiny amounts prevent these diseases. Once such conditions develop, however, it is necessary to use much larger amounts in order to eradicate them.

The concept that *very large quantities* of a vitamin, or of a part of a vitamin, would act in quite a different way was first discovered by a small group of men following a gradual development of the concept by my father, Dr. James Shute, and my brother, Dr. Evan Shute, and myself. Our basic idea was and is that very large quantities would act as a chemotherapeutic agent having a powerful effect on specific *degenerative* diseases. Today this concept is usually spoken of as the *therapeutic megavitamin approach to disease.*

To see this in proper perspective, it is necessary to refer to certain events in medical history.

Pasteur, Semmelweiss, Harvey, Jenner and others initiated the era in which bacterial infections and the conditions arising from them could be understood and dealt with. Over the years, methods have been developed to eliminate some of these hazards: vaccination, pasteurization, surgical cleanliness, antiseptics, sanitation techniques and the treatment of acute infections in the body with antibiotics.

The idea that resistance to a wide variety of infections, including some viral ones, might be increased and susceptibility to them thus decreased through the use of vitamins is more recent. Also recent is the idea of the usefulness of vitamins in combating degenerative diseases. This is a whole new medicine—new since the middle 1940s and growing rapidly and successfully!

Today, with some exceptions, modern medicine has pretty well conquered most infectious diseases. Its progress against degenerative diseases, by comparison, has been meager. I believe that with megavitamin therapy we stand on the edge of a great new era in which there are giant steps for the first time being taken in the treatment of the viral infections and degenerative diseases which now produce countless tragedies every year.

Vitamin E was isolated in 1922 by H.M. Evans and K.S. Bishop (2). In 1923, important work in the basic chemistry of Vitamin E was reported by B.J. Sure (3). My father's and my brother's concern with it began in 1933. Through work in obstetrics and gynecology and a research project based on this, they discovered that Vitamin E is an estrogen antagonist (a substance that neutralizes estrogen, the female sex hormone). Alpha tocopherol was synthesized in 1938 by P. Karrer and his associates (4) and became easily obtainable in synthetic form in 1941.

The importance of our bold conception of large-quantity vitamin therapy was suddenly dramatized in 1945 when a summer project, suggested by Dr. Evan Shute and carried out by a medical student named Floyd Skelton, resulted in the discovery of the beneficial effects of a very high daily dosage of pure alpha tocopherol in cardiovascular disease. Estrogen was given to dogs to induce thrombocytopenic purpura (a hemorrhaging disease). The disease was then cured with alpha tocopherol in many times the quantity usually given to patients up to that time. Finally, the disease was prevented in dogs with the use of the same substance.

Dr. Evan Shute had used what was then considered a

large dosage of a potent product of wheat germ oil to treat an acquaintance with severe angina pectoris in 1936. The result was excellent in this one case. However, I was unable to obtain similar results in hospitalized cardiac patients in the same year. We both forgot this until our interest was revived by the application of Skelton's research to a human patient with purpura whose cardiac symptoms were so severe that the surgeons and his attending physician were fearful that he would not survive an operation (the removal of the spleen).

Administration of 300 international units (IU) of synthetic alpha tocopherol—a dosage range worked out by Evan Shute and Skelton on the basis of the quantity used on the dogs—led to a rapid disappearance of congestive heart failure in this patient and to a slower resolution of his purpura.

Once more I joined in this clinical research, since I had a large group of cardiac patients in my practice while Evan, an obstetrician and gynecologist, had relatively few.

The alpha fraction of Vitamin E was isolated and identified in 1948 by Drs. K.L. Zierler, D. Grob and J.L. Lilienthal, Jr. (5). In the *American Journal of Physiology*, where they reported their findings, Zierler et al. state that it is a vigorous antithrombin and that it is antithrombic *in normal concentration* in the bloodstream. In treating patients who have suffered intravascular clotting, alpha tocopherol has since been shown to dissolve fresh clots in the veins. In those of patients subjected to major surgery, its ability to prevent embolism and thrombosis has also been demonstrated. In peripheral arteries it probably does this even more rapidly. And it does this *without interfering at all with the normal clotting mechanism* in cases of laceration or other forms of trauma.

It is clear, then, that alpha tocopherol must *not* be present in normal concentration in the bloodstreams of patients with coronary thrombosis and other conditions resulting from blood clots. But why? If blood remained fluid before 1912, what has happened in the meantime? Since the substance we are talking about is a vitamin, we must ask what has happened to our food to cause such a deficiency to exist in so many people.

There have been many changes in our environment since 1912: the multiplication of food additives, the removal of essential vitamins and minerals from food, the pollution of air, water and soil. But the greatest tragedy of all has been the removal of wheat germ from wheat, the stripping of flour and the "advances" that have been made in the manufacture of a basic staple food, bread. I am especially concerned with bread because this is the food which constitutes—or once constituted—our largest single source of natural Vitamin E.

The great biochemist, Dr. Roger Williams, writes that commercial "enriched" bread—our modern staple—is very low in nutrients. Dr. Williams (6) has reported an experiment in which he fed rats on nothing but this bread. Within three months, death from malnutrition had claimed 40 out of 64 rats, and the rest were severely stunted in their growth. In a second group of 64 rats, which he fed the same bread supplemented with additional nutrients, 61 were "alive and growing" at the end of the same period. Dr. Williams, speaking to the National Academy of Science, had words of praise for prepared cat and dog foods. "We feed our cats and dogs better than we do our children," he commented.

Few people know what is done to most bread before it reaches the grocery store. First of all, the wheat germ is removed and with it 87 percent of seven vitamins including Vitamin E, 84 percent of bulk minerals and 88 percent of trace metals. What is left is ground into flour which is then bleached. This removes any trace of Vitamin E which is left. Some Vitamin B_1 (thiamine) and Vitamin B_2 (riboflavin), niacin and iron are added and the flour is then termed "enriched." Incidentally, the iron added is sufficient to neutralize any Vitamin E that might still be there. (A better way to cut the growing incidence of anemia is to restore adequate amounts of Vitamin E to our diets and to correct hypothyroidism, a condition about which I shall have more to say as we proceed.)

Bread is not the only food which has been changed in this way over the years. It was reported in 1969 in the *Journal of Agriculture and Food Chemistry* that the alpha tocopherol content of whole maize, wheat, oats and rice goes down by as much as 90 percent when they are made into breakfast cereals. "Such cereals," says the report, "should be fortified to replace the loss. . . ."

Vitamin E has also been almost completely removed from refined hydrogenated oils, soy and cottonseed oil margarines, cottonseed oil, mayonnaise and other items of this kind. Many commercially deep-fried foods do not contain as much Vitamin E as they might because of freezing and storing procedures which cause losses of this vitamin. And today there are more than three thousand additives present in foods, many of which contribute to the destruction of the normal activity of Vitamin E.

Nutritionists today recognize that Vitamin E is essential in the diet. Unfortunately, however, many people in this field—and many others—still derive a false sense of security from the belief that the diet of the average person in the developed countries of the world is so rich in Vitamin E that deficiencies are unlikely. As recently as July-August 1973, an issue of *Nutrition Today* carried a long and, in many other respects, excellent article on Vitamin E which stated that "it is so prevalent in nearly every food man consumes it is quite unlikely that a vitamin E deficiency could arise."

The Food and Nutrition Board of the National Research Council (NRC) has estimated the adult requirement for alpha tocopherol to be between 20 and 30 IU per day. Because of changes in the processing of essential and basic foods over the last seventy years, it is very doubtful that many people today receive anything close to 30 IU per day, and surveys of Vitamin E levels in humans confirm that this must be a common situation. Typical diets in Great Britain, for example, have been estimated to contain less than 5 IU. Most commercial vitamin pills contain no Vitamin E. Many that do have a little also contain an iron compound that completely destroys the Vitamin E. There is none in most of the foods in the average American diet. Even in women, decreased intake of alpha tocopherol commonly depletes the stores of this important substance below the level effective in prevention.

Let me suggest that you pause for a moment now to consider the application of this information *in your own case*. Studies in the United States have also indicated a greatly reduced intake of Vitamin E, much of which is not the active part, the alpha portion. Most citizens obtain 5 to 8 IU per day in their diets—the minimum quantity the Food and Drug Administration (FDA) says infants should have! If a physician prescribes a diet rich in polyunsaturated fats, he is dropping the already marked deficiency of Vitamin E way below critical level. If you consume such a diet, it reduces the antithrombin in *your* bloodstream and thus encourages, produces or precipitates clots in blood vessels.

Little wonder, then, that I am so deeply concerned for the future of many apparently healthy individuals, as well as for that of those who have already had heart attacks! In fact, the current state of our nutrition—which is very often malnutrition—is the only valid explanation so far advanced for the growing epidemic of clots and resulting heart attacks, in that the progressive removal of alpha tocopherol from the human diet since the turn of the century exactly parallels the onset of coronary thrombosis and the increase in intravascular clotting in other areas of the body.

Later, in Chapter 8, I shall discuss another way in which it is now believed that myocardial infarction may occur—*without* an antecedent thrombus or clot in the larger coronary vessels. What I have to say about prevention and treatment, however,is equally applicable in this second type of situation since in this, as you will see, the myocardium dies because it is deprived of oxygen. And oxygen deprivation is a necessary consequence of a low level of alpha tocopherol in the bloodstream.

Alpha tocopherol, in fact, has been shown to have several other important effects on the individual cells of the body and on organs other than the heart. Actually, its value in the treatment and prevention of disease—alone or in combination with other vitamins and some of the amino acids and minerals that should be present in normal quantities in the human body—is just now beginning to be realized. Some of these will be mentioned in later chapters. Suffice it to say that alpha tocopherol therapy is changing many areas of medical treatment.

Little wonder, again, that I recommend megavitamin dosages of alpha tocopherol as the only means of restoring this essential substance in people whose bodies have been deficient in it for years!

REFERENCES

1. Cassidy, M. *British Medical Journal* 2, 782, 1946.
2. Evans, H.M. and Bishop, K.S. *Journal of Metabolic Research* 3, 233, 1923.
3. Sure, B.J. *Journal of Biological Chemistry* 74, 45, 1927.
4. Karrer, P., Escher, R., Fritsche, H., Keller, H., Ringier, B.H. and Salomon, H. *Helvetica Chimica Acta* 21, 939, 1938.
5. Zierler, K.L., Grob, D. and Lilienthal, Jr., J.L. *American Journal of Physiology* 153, 127, 1948.
6. Williams, R. *Nutrition Against Disease*. New York: Pitman, 1971.

4

VITAMIN E AS A VITAMIN

TWO GROUPS OF SCIENTISTS are involved in research on Vitamin E. There is, unfortunately, very little—if any—communication between members of these two factions.

One group is composed of professional researchers in physiology and biochemistry. Some of them are university teachers who do some research in addition to their teaching. Some are totally research-oriented. They use laboratory animals and follow the dictates of the NRC concerning recommended dietary requirements for Vitamin E: 5 IU for infants, 10 to 15 for children and 20 to 30 for adults. They adjust this dosage level to the sizes of their animal subjects. They study Vitamin E strictly as a vitamin—not as a therapeutic agent in the treatment of disease.

This group has been very productive. Its members have published many papers in scientific journals and have established the biochemical properties of Vitamin E—as a vitamin—in this dosage range. I usually think of their field of interest as "little e."

The other group consists mainly of clinicians, surgeons and others engaged in the practice of medicine who are using one of the tocopherols—alpha tocopherol—at megavitamin levels to treat humans. Dosages range from 75 to 100 IU a day for tiny premature infants with edema and hemolytic anemia to 2,000 to 3,200 IU for adult patients with cardiovascular or certain other kinds of disease. This group has also been very productive. They have turned out numerous papers which have been published in scientific journals throughout the civilized world. Their field of interest I call "Big E."

There is very little agreement between these two groups. Yet each makes important contributions to the advancement of science.

When I consider which is the more important of the two groups, I am reminded of something Albert Einstein once said in an address at the California Institute of Technology. "Concern for man himself and his fate," said Einstein, "must always form the chief interest of all technical endeavors, concern for the great unsolved problems . . . . " This wise remark from a very good and wise man confirms me in my instinctive preference for physicians who successfully treat people over laboratory workers with their rats, chickens, sheep, rabbits and monkeys.

This is not to minimize the usefulness of the laboratory group but merely to put their contributions into what I consider to be proper perspective. For I am about to embark now on a sketch of what the laboratory people have found out about Vitamin E and an outline of what clinicians have found and are applying in their work with patients. The latter will be the subject of the next chapter. The former I shall deal with now.

Just what, then, has the laboratory group to offer?

These scientists have thoroughly investigated the chemical structure of Vitamin E as a vitamin and have established its role in the normal biochemistry and physiology of animals and humans. They have firmly established that E is essential for the normal functioning of every cell in the human body. This was a necessary first step in overcoming the resistance to Vitamin E on the part of the U.S. Food and Drug people.

This piece of success has had considerable impact on our work. When we started using alpha tocopherol at megavitamin dosage levels, all bottles of the product had to carry on the label the statement that the need for Vitamin E in human nutrition had not been established. This changed in 1965 when the seventeenth revision of the U.S. Pharmacopeia included Vitamin E. Dr. Lloyd C. Miller, director of the revision, said that recent evidence compelled the recognition that "substantial quantities of this vitamin are essential to normal human nutrition." This, of course, was inevitable although long delayed. It is curious how a substance can be of no value one day and the next be declared essential to normal human nutrition!

Dr. Robert E. Hodges, Professor of Medicine at the University of California at Davis, has stated in an article in *Nutrah*, a publication of the American Heart Association, not only that "Vitamin E is an essential nutrient in the human diet" but also that "the need for Vitamin E is increased by a high intake of polyunsaturated fatty acids."

Dr. Hodges acknowledges that clinical evidence of deficiency may appear in persons who have some defect which limits their absorption of this vitamin. Unfortunately, he does not go on to comment upon the deficiencies that arise from insufficient intake and from individual variations in the absorption and excretion of the substance—what the great Dr. Roger J. Williams calls *biochemical individuality*.

Dr. Hodges also does not mention something that I think is of equal importance. This is the *type* of Vitamin E available in the individual's diet. Since alpha tocopherol is the most important member of the tocopherol group, it is important that the diet should contain this fraction. Wheat germ oil contains alpha and beta tocopherols; soybean oil contains alpha, gamma and delta tocopherols; cottonseed oil contains alpha and gamma forms; corn oil is rich in gamma tocopherol. But since only alpha tocopherol has, in sufficient strength, the characteristics that are needed in the treatment of disease, corn oil clearly contains only a relatively inert form of Vitamin E. Yet corn oil is the one, of all these fats, that we use most often. It appears in the majority of cooking oils and margarines.

Many physiologists and biochemists have added to our knowledge of the role of Vitamin E in the whole body, individual organs and individual cells. Dr. Jefferson N. Roehm and Dr. Luigi DeLuca, with their associates at the Massachusetts Institute of Technology, have produced evidence that Vitamin A and Vitamin E help maintain lung health and protect against air pollutants. As a result of experiments with mice, four researchers at Duke University Medical Center produced evidence in 1964 that explorers going into space should be fortified by a preliminary high dosage of Vitamin E. Finally, Dr. A.L. Tappel, Professor of Food Science, Technology and Nutrition at the University of California at Davis, has suggested that Vitamin E may slow the aging process. (Dr. Albert Barber, Professor of Zoology at the same institution, says that "there is reason to believe that Vitamin E may be helpful in slowing down the aging process," and a study by Dr. H.N. Marvin reveals that the "life span" of some body cells is lengthened by this vitamin.)

Dr. Tappel received the Borden Award in Nutrition in 1973. This Award recognizes distinctive research emphasiz-

ing the nutritional significance of any food or food compo-
nent. Tappel was cited for his important, innovative and
perceptive contributions relating to the mechanisms of lipid
peroxidation (the oxidation of fats) in biological systems and
to the factors that govern its occurrence and prevention.

He has related the potential consequences of these peroxidation reactions to biochemical processes in foods and to
cellular injury. The latter include the formation of age pig-
ments observed in certain pathological conditions, the activa-
tion of lysosomal (cell dissolving) enzymes in disease states
under particular nutritional and environmental conditions,
and lung damage from air pollution. The possibility of preventing these phenomena by understanding the role of Vitamin E and other antioxidants is a very important aspect of Dr.
Tappel's work.

In an article in the July-August 1973 issue of *Nutrition
Today*, Tappel states that Vitamin E's most important activity
takes place in the membranous parts of cells. "This is where
its real fascination lies," says Tappel, "for the clues to the
activity of Vitamin E within the cells suggest that we are
dealing with a substance of great potential."

He explains that within the membranous parts of cells,
Vitamin E interacts with the fatty substances (phospholipids,
cholesterol and triglycerides) that are their most important
constituents. Vitamin E apparently protects these substances
against destruction as a result of oxidation.

Tappel points out that Vitamin E acts in a similar way to
protect Vitamin A from oxidation and that it joins with Vitamin A in performing its function within the membranous
parts of the cells. Vitamin E also interacts, he says, with the
trace element selenium and with methionine and
cysteine-cystine, the sulfur amino acids. He also remarks on
the observed resemblance between the action of Vitamin E
and selenium.

Dr. Tappel comments that we now have a great deal of scientific data concerning the role of Vitamin E in nutrition and the effects of Vitamin E deficiency. "The very large number of symptoms that develop in Vitamin E-deficient animals indicates that this vitamin is very important to the function of most, if not all, of the tissues of the animal body."

On the subject of Vitamin E as a protection against damage to the lungs from air pollution, he states that since air pollution can produce damage to the lungs in the form of oxidation, "Vitamin E and the related protective systems now appear to be among the most important defensive systems. . . ."

Using rats, a number of researchers have investigated protection of the lungs by Vitamin E. It was discovered that the pollutants nitrogen dioxide and ozone can damage polyunsaturated fats within lung tissues by means of oxidation. It was also found that the animals could be protected against this damage by giving them large amounts of Vitamin E. Moreover, rats that had a Vitamin E deficiency suffered more damage from the ozone than rats that had received E beforehand. The research on nitrogen dioxide was done at the California State Department of Health, the work on ozone at the University of Southern California.

Dr. Tappel's article outlines this research and the extension of it at the Battelle Institute and the University of California at Davis. It is now known, because of this follow-up work, that rats suffer less damage from ozone, as well as nitrogen dioxide, if they are given Vitamin E in generous quantities. Vitamin E gave this protection both in the nutritional and in the therapeutic range. Dr. Tappel comments: "Since so many of the basic features of these animal tests are similar to conditions affecting some humans, it does not seem unwarranted to speculate about the application of these results to the human." This seems particularly significant in light of the fact that at Davis the pollutants were used in quantities adequate to simulate city smog on a bad day.

It is Dr. Tappel's view that because of Vitamin E's role as protector of polyunsaturated fats in the membranous parts of the cells, the need for this vitamin in the diet is related to dietary intake of these fats and the amounts of them already stored in the tissues. This, he says, is "a question of considerable importance to practicing physicians and dietitians in view of the emergent popularity of polyunsaturated fat food products."

People who are trying to avoid another coronary attack often are placed on diets in which there are more polyunsaturated than saturated fats. It would seem that these patients require an intake of Vitamin E that is commensurate with the amount of polyunsaturated fat they ingest. The amount, says Dr. Tappel, that has been offered as a guideline is 0.6 IU of Vitamin E per gram of polyunsaturated fats. People who have been on diets rich in polyunsaturates but who later go off them should realize that their need for this vitamin probably remains. Says Dr. Tappel: ". . . they still need to be concerned about the Vitamin E stabilization of the polyunsaturated fats stored in their adipose (fatty) tissues, since adipose tocopherol may be less efficiently stored than adipose polyunsaturated fats."

Later in this book, in Chapter 10, there is a diagram that shows the frightening application of this factor in the incidence of myocardial infarctions. The incidence rose slowly but steadily from 1912 to 1952, until cardiologists suddenly adopted the theory that decreasing the saturated and increasing the unsaturated or polyunsaturated fats in the diet was a possible way to prevent and treat coronary disease. As soon as this happened, there was a sudden rapid increase in the incidence of myocardial infarctions—and the increase continues to accelerate.

The relationship of Vitamin E to the actual quantity of polyunsaturated fats will be referred to several times in this book in relation to the epidemic of coronary disease and the unwise acceptance by cardiologists of the kind of diet that has just been mentioned.

Dr. Tappel says that Vitamin E is "one of the most hotly debated *nutritional* elements today." (Italics mine.) He goes on to state that there is a lack of agreement, even, that E is a vitamin and that it has been labeled "a vitamin in search of a disease"—this in a *Journal of the American Medical Association* editorial. (In contrast, there can be no such debate about the use of the alpha fraction at megavitamin levels in treating disease—here it is no longer "nutritional.")

Dr. Tappel traces the roots of the argument over the need for Vitamin E to the tendency of people to look for dramatic signs like cracked lips or bent backs as results of the absence of E. In fact, he says, "Vitamin E inadequacy is manifested in subtle and more diffuse ways, the most serious being the increased destruction by lipid peroxidation."

The same article also contains the suggestion that there should be more research into the effects of Vitamin E on the aging process. (It is believed that lipid peroxidation is closely connected with that process.)

5

A QUESTION OF QUANTITY

WHEN MY FATHER, my brother and I began giving our patients Vitamin E in relatively large doses back in the 1930s, we used what were then considered massive quantities of this substance in the form of a potent fresh wheat germ oil, cold pressed and kept refrigerated. To sustain pregnancies by combating abruptio placentae (premature detachment of the placenta from the wall of the uterus) my father and my brother Evan used quantities many times those which had ever been used before. And it was, similarly, with great quantities of wheat germ oil that in 1936 Evan successfully treated a patient with coronary insufficiency—the first case of cardiovascular disease to be approached in this way.

But wheat germ oil contains all the tocopherols—alpha, beta, gamma, delta, epsilon, eta and zeta—the entire Vitamin E complex. It was not until pure *alpha* tocopherol was first

56

produced synthetically in 1938 and then made available in 1941 that it was possible to use high levels of this especially potent fraction of the E complex at known strengths.

The first human patients treated with synthetic alpha tocopherol in large amounts were given 300 IU. This was ten times the maximum daily amount now listed by the NRC as the adult requirement. The results were dramatic and, in many cases, life-saving. There have actually never been better results in the more than 35,000 patients who have been treated by my father, my brothers, myself and the other doctors who later were associated with us in our work.

In 1950, Dr. Alton Ochsner and his group (1) reported that they had successfully repeated some work we had done earlier using alpha tocopherol to dissolve freshly formed clots in the veins of the legs. (This is a condition known as thrombophlebitis, or phlebitis for short, which is rapidly becoming more common following surgery, childbirth and trauma.) Ochsner et al. also reported that alpha tocopherol was successful in *preventing* phlebitis. For both treatment and prevention they used 600 IU a day—twenty times the recommended maximum today.

Since then, with increasing knowledge of the action of alpha tocopherol and the experience of treating thousands of patients, our dosage levels have risen—occasionally to as high as 3,200 IU a day or more than one hundred times the NRC's maximum.

Obviously we are using a vitamin in quantities that are in a totally different range than that contemplated by the NRC. This is because our purpose is entirely different from what they have in mind. We use Vitamin E not as a vitamin (something you take in small quantities to supplement the foods you eat) but as *a powerful chemotherapeutic agent in the treatment of disease.* Because they respond well or at least partially to alpha tocopherol, we are now able to treat a whole group of conditions heretofore untreatable or poorly dealt with, especially a number of degenerative diseases involving the cardiovascular system in its many anatomical areas.

The conditions in which we prescribe alpha tocopherol are all of them states in which one or another of the known characteristics of this versatile and unique substance can be expected, on a purely rational basis, to be helpful.

In this book, so far, I have dealt with only one of these characteristics: its ability to prevent the formation of the blood clots that are so often the cause of coronary thrombosis. As I have indicated just now, the same substance also has been shown to be effective against phlebitis. This is because in coronary thrombosis and phlebitis there is a common problem: a clotting mechanism that has somehow got out of control.

Vitamin E has several other known effects upon the body. It has the ability to perform five other important jobs:

- reduce the oxygen requirement of the tissues and cells;

- decrease abnormal capillary permeability (cut down the ability of blood cells and serum to pass through the walls of small blood vessels);

- function as a capillary vasodilator (produce enlargement of the small blood vessels);

- promote collateral circulation (stimulate development of alternate routes through which blood can travel if a primary route becomes blocked);

- promote epithelization (help form new skin).

I shall be telling you more about each of these functions in Chapter 7 and also in some of the later chapters in which I shall deal with particular disease states individually.

There are now in the world medical literature many hundreds of papers supporting the use of alpha tocopherol at megavitamin levels in treating a number of conditions related to difficulties of the types listed above. The following is a list of these and the number of supporting papers in each case.

- heart disease (132 papers);

- phlebitis (57 papers);

- complications of diabetes mellitus (46 papers);

- lack of blood supply to the extremities due to arteriosclerotic narrowing of their arteries (35 papers);

- Buerger's disease—narrowing of blood vessels to extremities with inflammation of the vessel lining and a marked tendency to clotting (13 papers);

- indolent ulcers—ulcers that seem unlikely to heal (60 papers);

- burns (30 papers).

There are applications in other fields as well: obstetrics and gynecology, ophthalmology and pediatrics, for example. Dermatology also contains a number of conditions in which Vitamin E has proved useful—conditions that were heretofore untreatable.

One of the earliest reports of this kind was that of Dr. H.D. Wilson (2) in 1964 in which he told of his successful treatment of epidermolysis bullosa dystrophica, a very unpleasant skin condition. In March 1973 a letter from Dr. Samuel Ayres, Jr. in *Current News in Dermatology* stated that Dr. Ayres and Dr. Richard Mihan had confirmed earlier (1950) results obtained by Dr. Milton Stout with alpha tocopherol in the treatment of another skin condition called pseudoxanthoma elasticum. Ayres and Mihan also reported successful treatment of epidermolysis bullosa with alpha tocopherol.

Ayres reported "gratifying results" with alpha tocopherol in the treatment of other skin conditions including Raynaud's phenomenon with gangrene, scleroderma, calcinosis cutis, Darier's disease, several types of cutaneous vasculitis, subcorneal pustular dermatosis, and benign chronic familial phemphigus. Some cases of chronic ulcers, discoid lupus erythematosis and granuloma annulare have also responded.

Dr. Ayres' letter to *Current News in Dermatology* reporting these results is reprinted in Appendix A by kind permission of the editor, Dr. Arthur G. Schoch.

My brother Evan's initial reports in the medical journals of the value of alpha tocopherol in treating threatened abortion have been supported by eighteen papers. There are fourteen papers supporting the use of alpha tocopherol in prevention of prematurity, nineteen on its role in the treatment of noneclamptic late toxemia (a type of blood poisoning that is a complication of pregnancy) and fifteen on dysmenorrhea (pain or difficulty in menstruating). On kraurosis (loss of skin elasticity) and senile vulvitis (inflammation of the external sex organs in older women) there are nine supporting papers. There are seven in the area of chronic cystic mastitis (an inflammation of the glandular tissue of the breast).

In ophthalmology, there have been reports of alpha tocopherol being helpful in treating such eye conditions as interstitial keratitis, diabetic retinitis, hypertensive retinopathy, retinal arteriospasm and macular degeneration. References to nine journal articles dealing with these and similar topics will be found in a separate list following the bibliographic references at the end of this chapter.

Alpha tocopherol has also been shown to be of value in

the treatment of edema (swelling) and hemolytic anemia (a condition in which red blood cells are destroyed) in premature infants. Drs. Ritchie, Fish, Grossman, and McMasters (3) reported in the *New England Journal of Medicine* in 1968 that among the infants they studied this condition was found to have associated with it a situation in which blood platelets are very numerous (thrombocytosis) and a low serum tocopherol level. "This syndrome," they wrote, "cleared completely in response to oral Vitamin E therapy."

In the mobile home park in Lake Worth, Florida, where I now spend part of the year is a seventy-year-old man who is very active athletically and one of the best shuffleboard players. For four or five years he had nocturnal leg cramps at least once a night, induced if he stretched his legs out. After his first month on E, he has not had a single cramp in two years.

The results in this case are not an isolated instance. The *Journal of the American Medical Association* in January 1972 published two letters dealing with the treatment of leg cramps with alpha tocopherol.

One letter, from Dr. Robert F. Cathcard III of San Mateo, California (4), referred to a 1969 paper by Samuel Ayres, Jr. and Richard Mihan (5) in which they reported the use of alpha tocopherol in the control of idiopathic night leg cramps. (Idiopathic is a word used to describe conditions whose cause or causes are unknown.) Dr. Cathcard says that he himself has treated almost one hundred patients with leg cramps and other types of idiopathic cramps and some with pain in the neck and lower part of the back with 300 IU of alpha tocopherol. He states: "I would second Ayres and Mihan's observation that massive doses of tocopherol (alpha) are extremely effective in the control of idiopathic night cramps."

The other letter (6) is from Drs. Ayres and Mihan. It notes that their series of twenty-six nocturnal leg cramp cases included "restless legs" syndrome and rectal cramps. Alpha tocopherol had given "satisfactory relief in all cases." A further series of seventy-six cases, they said, had included some with restless legs and rectal cramps and one athlete training for the Olympics whose work in running, swimming and weight lifting had been followed by severe cramps. They conclude by saying: "All of these patterns received prompt and gratifying relief from the oral administration of Vitamin E (d-alpha tocopherol acetate)."

The publication of these two letters elicited a wry comment from the editor of another medical journal. He suggested that had the subject of these letters been anything other than Vitamin E it would have warranted a complete major paper!

It should be mentioned that Ritchie et al., working with tiny premature infants, used 75 to 100 IU of alpha tocopherol per day, which is a megavitamin level for such babies. In fact, it is fifteen to twenty times the 5 IU recommended dietary allowance of the NRC. Ayres and Mihan, in treating leg cramps, used 300 to 400 IU daily, occasionally 800. Ayres states that in the skin conditions he mentioned they have usually prescribed alpha tocopherol in doses of 400 to 800 IU per day. In some cases, he says, they have prescribed up to 1,600 or 2,000 IU per day.

Dr. Ayres adds that he has encountered no untoward side-effects. However, if a patient has severe hypertension, serious cardiac impairment, or is a diabetic on insulin, Dr. Ayres recommends that physicians should start him on "much smaller doses such as 100 IU daily, which can be gradually increased over a period of weeks or several months."

I shall go into the matter of dosage and hazards of this kind in more detail in Chapter 16.

The Shute concept that vitamins might be used in therapeutic doses to deal with hitherto hard-to-treat illnesses has also led to the use of other vitamins or portions of them in this way. Over the years, the megavitamin approach has been successfully extended to the treatment of schizophrenia, resistant allergies, virus infections, many dermatological problems and many, many other conditions.

Dr. Fred Klenner, Dr. Constance Spittle and many others have done extensive investigation into the therapeutic value of ascorbic acid (Vitamin C) in doses of one to five thousand milligrams (mg) daily. Dr. Spittle has demonstrated a reduction by 50 percent in the incidence of post-surgical thrombophlebitis through the use of large amounts of Vitamin C. Dr. Klenner has shown the value of Vitamin C in acute allergic reactions to insect stings and in a wide variety of conditions involving the cardiovascular system. This is not surprising since Vitamin C, like Vitamin E, is an antioxidant (though a water-soluble one). His most important discovery, however, has been the fact that Vitamin C is a potent therapeutic agent in otherwise intractable virus infections.

At a 1973 meeting of the International College of Applied Nutrition, a veterinarian presented a paper on the use of intravenous ascorbic acid in the huge quantities first recommended by Dr. Klenner. The purpose, in veterinary medicine, is the treatment in dogs of a deadly virus disease, distemper. By the time dogs with this disease reach the veterinarian, there is usually little hope of recovery. Of those that survive, many are blind, deaf or both. Yet recovery is the rule with 5½ gm of ascorbic acid intravenously followed by oral administration, and these dogs do not go deaf or blind. The results are so excellent that this veterinarian no longer hospitalizes the dogs. He simply gives the intravenous C and sends the dog and the appropriate amount of oral C home with the owner.

Dr. Abraham Hoffer has been using megavitamin therapy, along with some traditional methods, in the treatment of early schizophrenia. He has had more recoveries and fewer recurrences than are usual among such patients when treated by conventional methods. In the United States he has acquired many co-workers and converts, in his native Canada little but criticism!

Dr. Alan Cott has been using megavitamin therapy with success in treating children who are hyperkinetic (overactive) and who have learning defects or disabilities.

Twelve years ago very few doctors were interested in hypoglycemia (low blood sugar). Now all that has changed. Two active organizations with rapidly increasing memberships are devoted chiefly, though not exclusively, to hypoglycemia. Patients with this condition are now being treated successfully with diet plus three essential vitamins, including 800 IU daily of Vitamin E.

It is easy to demonstrate the unique effectiveness of Vitamin E. It doesn't take a highly trained medical specialist. Any intelligent doctor can do it—and many have done so. All that's needed is one case, if it is the kind of condition in which there has never before been even one single successful instance of treatment by traditional methods. One case, as we have seen, was all that Milton Stout presented before the Los Angeles Dermatological Society, yet Samuel Ayres, Jr. refers to it in his *Current News* letter as "this astounding therapeutic accomplishment."

A salesman for a company that manufactures Vitamin E ointment once told me a story. And this tale has a certain pure scientific beauty to it. One spring day he acquired a severe sunburn while building a barbecue in his backyard. After dinner, he realized how badly burned he was and he started to apply the ointment, knowing that it was uniquely effective in treating sunburn. Suddenly he stopped, realizing that here was a chance to demonstrate to his doubting medical clientele along the west coast just what E could do. He began applying the ointment again, but confined it to *half* of the burned area. The next day there was no sign of sunburn on the half on which he had used the ointment but blisters as large as fifty-cent pieces all over the other half. He spent the week visiting his medical skeptics—a most successful week.

This story offers very dramatic proof of the efficacy of alpha tocopherol treatment. And the fact that this salesman proved his point—on his own burn—by using the ointment on only half of it serves to remind me of the discussion which has surrounded the nonperformance, by my brother Evan and myself, of what are called "controlled" studies—the kind of experiments which some of our critics have maintained are necessary to prove the effectiveness of alpha tocopherol therapy in the treatment of certain conditions.

Controlled studies, of course, are ones in which the results of a new treatment in one group of subjects are compared either with those of some standard treatment or with those of a placebo or with those of nontreatment, in another group of subjects. If the subjects do not know to which group they have been assigned, such a study is also referred to as being "single-blind." If the experimenters themselves also do not know until afterward which individuals have been assigned to which group, such a study is called "double-blind."

The object of all this is to provide a clear basis for comparison between the results of two different procedures or courses of action. Nevertheless, I have many reservations concerning the various types of controlled studies.

First of all, it is possible for their results to be misleading. In the early days of Vitamin E therapy, for example, several experiments were conducted which demonstrated that it was of no clinical value. The workers who did these experiments did not know that the product they were using contained only about one-seventh the quantity of active principle that they believed it to contain. Also, their tests were run for a relatively short time. They were terminated before an experimenter today would expect to see the effects. Yet these studies proved to a great many doctors, and cardiologists in particular, that Vitamin E was valueless.

Drugs are often difficult to study in this way unless the proper dosage is known beforehand. Moreover, some drugs—while of the utmost value when used correctly—can be dangerous when improperly used. And whether a drug is being used properly in a group of subjects can depend not only on knowing what dosage is generally correct but on making allowances for the marked biochemical individuality which can affect a subject's response to a potent medication.

Had digitalis, a most useful substance in treating some forms of heart disease, been subjected to a study in which the same dosage was given to a large number of patients, it would very likely have been thrown out at the outset. Digitalis works only within the specific dosage range appropriate to the individual patient. In subminimal levels it is virtually useless, and in overdosage it can kill.

Think, too, of the fate of insulin had it been subjected to such a double-blind controlled study. Here, the correct dosage level in the individual patient may vary as much as one to twenty. It would be very simple, in fact, using the knowledge we now have, to devise double-blind controlled studies that would prove insulin useless, useful, or extremely dangerous.

Where exactly the same treatment is to be given to all the subjects in one group in a double-blind experiment, considerations of biochemical individuality cannot be attended to. If Vitamin E is being studied, for instance, a patient whose condition might improve if his dosage were increased will not have the benefit of the increase so long as the study continues in strict accordance

Where exactly the same treatment is to be given to all the subjects in one group in double-blind experiment, considerations of biochemical individuality cannot be attended to. If Vitamin E is being studied, for instance, a patient whose condition might improve if his dosage were increased will not have the benefit of the increase so long as the study continues in strict accordance with this plan.

A further criticism of such an experiment would be concerned with patients who were not to be given Vitamin E. Our feelings and beliefs in this area would make it impossible for us to deny the benefits of alpha tocopherol therapy to patients who, in our view, would benefit from it—even if the purpose were to provide the kind of proof which seems to be demanded by a great many people.

We believe, in fact, that more controlled studies are done than are necessary, In many cases, all that is required is to make a comparison of the results of a good treatment such as alpha tocopherol therapy with the known course of a given disease—its mortality rate, the eventual cause of death, its total prognosis. Medical history provides a number of examples of the adoption of successful treatments on the basis of this type of evidence. The first really successful treatment of leprosy was rapidly adopted without a single control and after but a few obvious responses to the new therapy. Vaccination, inoculation for diphtheria and scarlet fever, insulin, the antiseptics, and chlorination—modalities of treatment which have conquered many of the most feared epidemics of the past—also were not subjected to controlled studies. It seems to me, therefore, that our use of comparison between the results of alpha tocopherol therapy and the known courses of a number of diseases has, in itself, produced results which are sufficiently convincing. Fortunately, the worship of the god of double-blind controlled experiment is of relatively recent origin.

Let me summarize very simply by saying that considerations of this kind—along with many years of clinical experience in the use of alpha tocopherol in therapeutic doses —have led me to regard this therapy as being of proven value in the treatment of a wide variety of conditions.

Over the years we have achieved substantial relief in 80 to 85 percent of our more than thirty-five thousand cardiovascular patients!

REFERENCES

1. Ochsner, A., DeBakey, M.E. and DeCamp, P.T. *Journal of the American Medical Association* 144, 831, 1950.
2. Wilson, H.D. *Canadian Medical Association Journal* 90, 1315, 1964.
3. Ritchie, J.H., Fish, M.B., Grossman, M. and McMasters, V. *New England Journal of Medicine* 279, 1185, 1968.
4. *Journal of the American Medical Association* 219, 216, 1972.
5. Ayres, S., Jr. and Mihan, R. *California Medicine* 111, 87, 1969.
6. *Journal of the American Medical Association* 219, 216, 1972.

FURTHER REFERENCES (OPHTHALMOLOGY)
(In chronological order)

Stone, S. *Archives of Ophthalmology* 30, 467, 1943. (Interstitial keratitis.)

Carreros, R.J. *Prensa Medica Argentina* 37, 1764, 1947. (Keratoconus.)

Dominguez. D.D. *Presse Medicale* 58, 972, 1950. (Retinal degeneration and myopic chorioretinitis.)

Terzani, G. *Policlinica Sezione Pratica* 58, 1381, 1951. (Diabetic retinitis. Incidental improvement in other aspects of patients' cardiovascular systems.)

Seidenar, R., Mars, G. and Morpurgo, M. *Acta Gerontologica* 1, 55, 1951. (Arteriosclerotic hypertensive retinopathy.)

Cameron, A.J. *Medical Press* 144, 543, 1952. (Hypertensive retinitis.)

Zampetti, C.A. *Proceedings of the Third International Congress on Vitamin E, September, 1955.* (Retinal artery spasm.)

Raverdino, E. *Proceedings of the Third International Congress on Vitamin E, September, 1955.* (Macular degeneration of vascular origin.)

Johuda, H.M. *Journal of Clinical Ophthalmology* 17, 797, 1963. (Central serous chorioretinitis.)

6

CONFLICT AND SUPPORT

IT MAY SEEM STRANGE TO YOU—as it does to me
—that the two groups we have been discussing should engage in very little communication with one another. It will
appear even more puzzling, I am sure, when I come to describe in this chapter the actual hostility to the clinical investigators which has been demonstrated by the basic science
group. All I can deduce is that somewhere along the line the
latter have been encouraged to cooperate with some agencies
apparently bent on suppressing the rapid spread of correct
and effective alpha tocopherol megavitamin therapy among
doctors and the knowledge of its success among the laity.

To me, it appears that the prime reasons behind all this go
back a good many years. Our basic findings have been reported to medical groups, including the Kansas City
Academy of Medicine in 1947 and the Ontario Medical Association in 1953. However, the American Medical Associa-

tion in 1955 first accepted a presentation by us for its Annual
Convention, then cancelled it. This may have been the result
of pressure from some individuals or group within its membership. Having taken this action, the Association subsequently took a stand against us, and has avoided publiciz-
ing any evidence contrary to their stand, which might be in-
terpreted that they were wrong in so vital a matter.

Over the years this evidence, starting as a trickle, has
grown to a deluge. Many curious incidents have occurred as a
result.

The Association's official organ, the *Journal of the American Medical Association*, for example, published in 1950 what
was really a full confirmation of our basic claims when it
printed Ochsner's article(1) on the treatment of phlebitis with
alpha tocopherol (while at the same time denouncing in an
editorial the pioneers of this approach as quacks and charla-
tans). Is is possible that this slipped by because he used the
words "alpha tocopherol" instead of Vitamin E"? (This
editorial confusion may possibly have persisted. In the
Journal's Question and Answer column, authorities have several times over the years mentioned the application of alpha
tocopherol in the treatment of human pathological conditions.) But it is our guess that the *Journal* has never forgiven
Dr. Ochsner, since his subsequent papers have been published elsewhere, in the *New England Journal of Medicine* and
Postgraduate Medicine, for example.

For doctors whose work has been denounced so
thoroughly in such a prestigious publication, some of the
other "press" we have had has not been too bad. Over the
years interest in Vitamin E has grown and public knowledge
and understanding of its value have accumulated, thanks in
part to some of the helpful and accurate books and articles
that have appeared.

Interest in E has mounted slowly since the publication in

1954 of our first book, *Alpha Tocopherol (Vitamin E) in Cardiovascular Disease* (2), and the subsequent appearance of a version of this prepared for laymen, *Your Heart and Vitamin E* (3). Momentum has come, also, from the influence of our patients and that of the ever-increasing number of doctors who have tried Vitamin E for themselves and found that it helped their patients too. Patients, in turn, have formed the nuclei of widening circles of friends who could see the improvement in their condition.

For quite a few years, also, *Prevention* magazine has carried information on the usefulness and effectiveness of Vitamin E treatment. Its first owner and editor, the late J. I. Rodale, was one of the first patients seen after the opening of the Shute Institute for Laboratory and Clinical Medicine in London, Ontario, Canada in 1949. This magazine has a very large readership of people interested in their health, in preventing disease and avoiding "disaster medicine."

The reception of our work among doctors and laymen alike has improved most markedly, however, in the past ten years. In 1964 a medical writer named Herbert Bailey wrote a book entitled *Vitamin E, Your Key to a Healthy Heart* (4). This has sold thousands of copies to date and is in its eleventh printing. This book gave the factual story of Vitamin E and its vicissitudes. Following its success, five or six other writers have published books on Vitamin E for the popular market—most of them, in my opinion, pretty inadequate. Finally, in the late 1960s, Harald Taub, Managing Editor of *Prevention*, suggested that it was time for the publication of a new book on the subject by a physician—ideally, one closely associated with the beginnings of Vitamin E therapy. Since there is no one in this whole wide world who has seen the number of cardiovascular patients that I have seen and, of course, no one who has treated so many of them with alpha tocopherol, I was the logical one to do it. The result was the publication in 1969 of *Vitamin E for Ailing and Healthy Hearts* (5) with Harald Taub.

Reception of this book has been most interesting. Partly owing to its bibliography of some 125 of the seven hundred papers confirming the value of alpha tocopherol in the field of cardiovascular disease, and partly owing to its case histories illustrating the results obtained with alpha tocopherol and alpha tocopherol alone in cases in which there was otherwise no help, the book opened the eyes of those physicians who were curious enough to read it because of their own interest or at the suggestion of patients.

As a result of the publication of this book, we have had many requests for specific information from doctors, including several certified specialists in cardiology. Last year's correspondence with this group alone fills three bulging folders!

But physicians, of course, have not been our only readers. The sale of the book in hard cover was phenomenal, and it continues to sell now that it is available in paperback. Of course, each book sold has alerted more than one person through family and friends. It would appear that there are now very few people who do not know first hand or have not heard of someone who has received worthwhile help through alpha tocopherol therapy. This is owing, in part, to our long record of success in treating patients and our very great numbers of patients and the number and variety of places from which they have come: from every state in the United States, from every province in Canada and from Australia, New Zealand, Ceylon, England, Ireland, Switzerland and Italy. I think that it is also partly owing to the favorable publicity we have sometimes enjoyed and to the effectiveness of the book.

There is also much indirect evidence of the snowballing acceptance of alpha tocopherol therapy. The media have registered their amazement. *Business Week* (20 November 1971) contains an article entitled "Riding the Vitamin E Boom." Comments this publication: "Suddenly this year, people are popping Vitamin E again like mad . . . . That's why mutual funds are jostling each other to get shares of R.P. Scherer Corp." *Business Week* goes on to explain that Scherer has about 75 percent of the world market in the type of capsules used to contain liquid vitamins and certain other pharmaceuticals.

An article by Robert Vare, ("All About Vitamin E," *Cosmopolitan* magazine, November 1972) estimates that "as many as twenty million of us take E regularly and millions more get it with other vitamins in composite pills." (I have pointed out elsewhere that the amounts contained in such composites are very small by my standards, but Vare's point is nevertheless very good. Inclusion of E in such pills at least illustrates the fact that a lot of people are now aware of it.)

Articles on Vitamin E have been appearing in other unexpected places. For example, *Moneysworth*, a consumer newsletter, printed an article entitled "Now, The Vitamin E Craze" in its 27 May 1972 issue. "Americans," it said, "are gobbling Vitamin E capsules the way kids guzzle gumdrops . . . ." *Moneysworth* goes on to state that the pharmaceutical industry is "understandably ecstatic" and that some retailers have seen a marked jump in sales of Vitamin E since 1969. The newsletter even quotes a comment on the phenomenon from the *Wall Street Journal!*

A Canadian distributor of Vitamin E products not long ago produced files that showed that he received regular orders from 1,180 doctors who buy their supplies directly from him. From a similar company in California some seven thousand doctors buy Vitamin E directly. At recent meetings of the International Academy of Preventive Medicine—an organization that I shall tell you more about in Chapters 10 and 18—a show of hands demonstrates that at least three-quarters of the members are using E, and I remember that very few of them were doing so when I first addressed them a few years ago.

All this favorable reaction has not gone unnoticed by the

opposition. An early evidence of concern was the appearance of an unfavorable review of my book, *Vitamin E for Ailing and Healthy Hearts*, in the *New England Journal of Medicine*. (This is the same journal which on 23 July 1964 published a letter from Dr. Ochsner stating that he had "for a number of years . . . routinely prescribed alpha tocopherol . . . . " and that it is "a potent inhibitor of thrombin . . . and a safe prophylactic against venous thrombosis.") The majority of the "scare" articles that have appeared, however, have been written by nutritionists or nonpracticing physicians who usually prefer to remain anonymous. For example, a lengthy treatment in the January 1973 issue of *Consumer Reports* was anonymous.

A statement that I feel I should single out for reply here is the one attributed in the Vare article to Dr. Frederick J. Stare, Chairman of Harvard's Department of Nutrition: "Not one single reputable physician thinks that Vitamin E is worth a damn for anything. I don't know of any illness in the United States which has ever been cured by the vitamin. Nor do I know of any disease that results from a lack of it."

This is not the first nor the last pronouncement of this nutritionist to discredit megavitamin E therapy. He has used his widely syndicated newspaper column to bring up the subject only to condemn it on numerous occasions. Of course, Dr. Stare is wrong in his belief. Many reputable physicians —not theoretical nutritionists—are using this therapy with excellent results obtainable no other way.

Dr. Alton Ochsner, head of the Ochsner Clinic in New Orleans—the "little Mayos of the South"—is one of the three most honored surgeons in America. He says that Vitamin E is a potent antithrombin and will dissolve fresh clots in the veins of the extremities and will prevent their formation in risk cases. In a paper entitled "Preventing and Treating Venous Thrombosis" which was presented before the fifty-second annual assembly of the Interstate Postgraduate Medical Association and published in 1968 in the journal *Postgraduate Medicine* he states: "In addition, for 15 years I have used alpha tocopherol routinely in the treatment of patients who have been subjected to trauma of any magnitude. None of these patients have had pulmonary embolism. Tocopherol in the presence of calcium acts as an antithrombotic agent; only the alpha tocopherol has this property. It does not produce a hemorrhagic tendency and can be used safely. The physicians in our department of urology use it in treating patients who have had transurethral resection."

Drs. Ayres and Mihan published an account of the successful treatment of leg cramps and "restless legs" syndrome in 1969. Samuel Ayres, Jr. is Emeritus Clinical Professor of Medicine (Dermatology) at the University of California at Los Angeles (The Center for Health Sciences). Richard Mihan is Assistant Clinical Professor of Medicine (Dermatology and Syphilology) at the University of Southern California School of Medicine. They have used Vitamin E in the treatment of several dermatological conditions and have presented papers on this work before the American College of Physicians, the American Dermatological Association and the Pacific Dermatological Association.

Joshua H. Ritchie, M.D., Mathews B. Fish, M.D. and Moses Grossman, M.D. presented a paper at an annual meeting of the Society for Pediatric Research and at meetings of the Western Society for Clinical Research and the Western Society for Pediatric Research. This paper, as I have already noted, was published in the *New England Journal of Medicine* in 1968. They stated that they had successfully treated premature infants with widespread edema and anemia with Vitamin E (in our dosage range, please note).

There are many, many more doctors of medicine in the United States and throughout the world—doctors as entitled to recognition and respect as are Ochsner, Ayres, Mihan, Fish and Grossman—who have used Vitamin E to cure and to treat abnormal conditions in humans.

Such statements as Dr. Stare's deserve censure for their sweeping generalities which may hinder development of a treatment which is safe in most, but not all, cases and extremely successful in prolonging lives, saving legs from amputation and obviating in many burn cases the necessity for skin grafting, recurrent pain and prolonged hospitalization.

Dr. Robert E. Olson of the St. Louis University School of Medicine presented a paper on Vitamin E at the Annual Scientific Meeting of the American Heart Association in 1972. This paper was released to the press and widely disseminated. It was reported in the press that Olson had stated that there was no evidence that large daily doses of Vitamin E could help anyone's heart. He was quoted, however, as stating that the only proven clinical use of Vitamin E was in the treatment of intermittent claudication. Now this is a condition so completely analogous to the common conditions in the heart that are caused by abnormalities in the coronary artery blood supply that if Vitamin E works for intermittent claudication it simply *must* also work for coronary insufficiency!

The authors mentioned in this chapter as having published articles supporting Vitamin E therapy are merely representative of the many who have published their results in the treatment of human disease conditions with alpha tocopherol at megavitamin levels. Professor A.M. Boyd of the University of Manchester (England), Dr. H.T.G. Williams in Canada and lately Dr. Knüt Haeger of Sweden are impressive names in high places—all persons whose papers deserve to be considered even by Dr. Stare.

In the past few years the basic science group has held a number of "international symposia on Vitamin E." At one that was held by the New York Academy of Sciences in 1971 it was reported in *Medical World News* (24 December 1971) that for two days "international investigators" discussed the nutritional muddle but could come to no agreement concerning Vitamin E's exact role in cellular metabolism. We heard of this by chance, after its program had been arranged. We did not attend because there were no papers of interest to us—that is, none that we considered to be of practical clinical value.

In June 1973 *Nutrition Today* carried a notice concerning another of these meetings. This one was to be known as the "International Symposium on Vitamin E, Minneapolis, September 26-27." The notice said that information could be obtained by writing to Dr. M.K. Horwitt at the Department of Biochemistry, St. Louis University School of Medicine. I wrote to Dr. Horwitt (29 June 1973) requesting information and asking if I could arrange to have an area adjacent to the meetings for a continuous presentation of a representative selection of our colored slides.

The slides I refer to show the results of the treatment of acute thrombophlebitis, chronic varicose ulcerations, various ulcers, diabetic gangrene and other conditions. Not one of the cases presented in them had responded to what has heretofore been considered to be the "correct" treatment. These slides have been responsible for the "conversion" of many doctors in the California area and more recently for that of the majority of the members of the International Academy of Preventive Medicine and the International Academy of Metabology, and have strengthened the stand taken many years ago by the International College of Applied Nutrition. I thought it was only reasonable that since they establish the efficacy of megavitamin alpha tocopherol beyond any doubt, such a presentation would be enthusiastically received by the sponsors of the "International Symposium on Vitamin E."

NOT SO!

Dr. Horwitt replied (6 July 1973) that the number of

participants would be very limited and that "Only speakers and discussants who have recently conducted controlled experiments on the biochemistry and physiology of the tocopherols have been invited." He also indicated that there would be no booths. I replied (8 July 1973) that an "international symposium on Vitamin E" should have a broader focus. All interested scientists—physicians as well as biochemists and physiologists—should be accommodated. Finally (1 August 1973) Dr. Horwitt refused me: "I regret that it would defeat our purpose to invite you to our symposium."

Even so, one paper of considerable clinical significance was presented at this "International Symposium on Vitamin E." Somehow Dr. Knüt Haeger from the General Hospital at Malmo, Sweden was allowed to present his work on the treatment of intermittent claudication with Vitamin E. This was a controlled trial described in *Vascular Diseases* (6). In that experiment, twelve legs were amputated, only one belonging to a patient in the alpha tocopherol-treated group which represented 104 out of 227 subjects in the study. I shall describe this study in some detail in Chapter 11.

Medical people generally have had to accept Haeger's study as definitive. And this leaves some of them with a real problem. How can a substance work to support and save ischemic tissue (tissue lacking a proper blood supply) in one area of the body and not have the slightest effect on exactly the same situation in other parts of the body? Curious, too, is the fact that Dr. Haeger's paper seemed convincing when the same observations made by the Shutes and confirmed by Professor Boyd of the University of Manchester and in some thirty-one other papers failed to impress these same scientists. (Dr. Boyd reported success in the treatment of 1,345 patients with this condition in 1963 and his work includes a report on a controlled series.)

Obviously, after twenty-seven years of noncommunication between the basic science group and the clinical medicine group (little e and Big E), communication between the two groups is impossible. To quote Dr. Horwitt, the biochemists, physiologists and nutritionists "try to avoid thinking in terms of 'cures' but [strive] to obtain basic physiological data which may someday be useful." At this date such a statement is palpably ludicrous. People in clinical medicine who have come to know the effectiveness of alpha tocopherol in relieving human suffering and lengthening lives find it difficult to retain such detachment.

The Shute brothers do not maintain this detachment. Because they do not, there are several thousand people who have been directly helped, and who knows how many more thousands the world over who have been helped as a result of our work. We accepted Dr. Boyd's results as confirming ours some ten years before the acceptance of Haeger's work.

At this point I cannot resist sharing with you the most recent episode in Dr. Fredrick Stare's campaign against Vitamin E. He has a syndicated newspaper column in which he frequently states his position on the subject of Vitamin E therapy—one of complete and absolute condemnation. However, he has now had to admit, though ever so reluctantly, that "there are suggestions that large amounts of Vitamin E may help alleviate the situation" known as intermittent claudication, though he hastens to add, "but there is very little sound evidence that it does."

You will remember that Dr. Robert E. Olson was widely quoted as saying that Vitamin E had no value in any cardiovascular condition—*except intermittent claudication*. This has put Dr. Stare in a difficult position since Olson is a fellow "nutritionist," a pupil and a friend. Note the contrast in two of Stare's columns, one week apart.

A column was published under his name in *The Vancouver Sun*, for 10 July 1974 headed "Vitamin E Use Under

Attack." In it he comments on two letters in *The Lancet*—one by Dr. M.H. Briggs of Australia and a later one by Dr. Sven Dahl of Sweden, and an article from Edinburgh (reference not given). The concluding paragraph of the column contains this statement: "There is no evidence, T.V. shows to the contrary, that any known illness of man is helped by extra Vitamin E, and there is increasing evidence that extra Vitamin E taken by so many gullible individuals may do harm."

Just one week later, his column carried an interesting question and answer—on the subject of Vitamin E—though Vitamin E was not headlined this time. The headline, rather, was "Pasteurized Milk Is Safe." Here is the question and answer in full.

Q. Dr. Robert E. Olson, Professor of biochemistry and medicine at St. Louis University was recently quoted in the papers as saying that the only type of disease found to benefit from large doses of Vitamin E is a cardiovascular ailment known as intermittent claudication. Does this disease affect the circulation of leg arteries, making walking difficult and painful?

A. Dr. Olson is a good friend, a former student and staff member of Harvard's department of nutrition and a bright physician who is very knowledgeable in nutrition. He has also done considerable basic research on Vitamin E. You are right in that a condition known as intermittent claudication is occasionally responsible for pain in the lower legs, particularly during walking. There are suggestions that large amounts of Vitamin E may help alleviate this situation, but very little sound evidence that it does.

Is this a tiny crack in the position of the world's Number One opponent of Vitamin E therapy?

Near the opening of this chapter I outlined the growth in public awareness of alpha tocopherol and its effectiveness that has taken place since 1954. Following that, I gave you some idea of the positions taken by some of the skeptics in the "opposition." Now let me conclude by telling you of a couple of pleasant encounters I've had recently with investigators from abroad.

We have known for many years that the clinical use of alpha tocopherol is world-wide. My brother Evan keeps a constant watch on the world medical literature in our field in order to prepare summaries of it for publication in the journal of the Shute Foundation, the nonprofit organization that operates the Shute Institute. (This journal, called simply *The Summary*, goes to many interested physicians and to medical libraries throughout the world—some twelve thousand copies per issue.) We also hear from patients living in many countries, and we receive letters from physicians all over the civilized world who are interested in and using Vitamin E.

Recently I was privileged to be a speaker at a medical convention in Las Vegas. On the same program was Dr. Hans Nieper from Germany. He is the authority, having done most of the original work, on the orotates—the magnesium and sodium salts of orotic acid. On an occasion when we were both on a panel discussing coronary heart disease, he corroborated my answers to the questions on alpha tocopherol treatment from the doctors in the audience. To my delight, he seemed very much surprised that there was any longer any question in anyone's mind about its efficacy in cardiovascular disease.

On Dr. Nieper's return to Germany he sent me a reprint of an article (in German) by von Rave et al. (7) showing that mesenchyme metabolism accelerations caused by toxin stimulation can be met by large Vitamin E doses and also that

proliferation of granulation tissue (new tissue formed in healing) is diminished. "These findings," say the authors, "confirm clinical and other experimental observations that Vitamin E has a favorable effect in a great number of connective
tissue diseases." This, of course, confirms our many observations since using alpha tocopherol in this way. What interested me most was the bibliography. Forty-three scientific
papers were quoted!

Shortly afterward I received an invitation to present a
paper at a medical conference in Baden-Baden, Germany on
the subject of coronary artery disease. Unfortunately I had to
refuse because I had already accepted an invitation to present
our work, in three parts, at a medical-dental meeting in
Hawaii. I mention this to illustrate the world-wide interest in
and acceptance of our work and to remind the reader that the
majority of the clinical investigation into the effects of Vitamin
E has been a direct result of our original reports.

Not too long ago, we had a visit from Lady Phyllis
Cilento, a doctor from Australia and the wife of another
doctor, Sir Raphael Cilento, head of the Public Health Service
in that country. (The Cilentos have two sons and a daughter
who are also physicians and a daughter, Diane, who is a
well-known actress.)

Three circumstances in Lady Cilento's work in Australia
both interested her and bothered her. First, she had had some
practical experience in the use of alpha tocopherol to soften
scar tissue and had seen its effects in restoring circulation to
dead-looking toes. Secondly, she had become disturbed by
the increasing number of deaths from coronary occlusions
and the disablement of those who survived such attacks.
Thirdly, she had searched the literature on Vitamin E and
found it to be voluminous—yet ignored by some investigators.

This indomitable woman decided to "go in search of the
truth about Vitamin E." And so she set out on a long journey

that brought her to our door, among others.

In many countries she found doctors who were using Vitamin E successfully: one practicing in Singapore; a leading heart specialist in Bavaria, Germany; one in England who had visited the Shute Institute and returned home to begin the use of E. This English physician told Lady Cilento that Vitamin E did all that we had claimed for it. "There is no doubt that it improves the circulation," he told her. "Those with angina pectoris find that they can do much more without chest pain, and in my hands those who have survived a coronary thrombosis do not suffer a second attack."

In Canada she went to research centers and then had a long visit with me and my brother Evan. Lady Cilento also took time to see Dr. Lambert, the noted Irish veterinarian who has done much work with E, and to tour the stud farm in Canada which has used Vitamin E to improve the performances of their brood mares and stallions and particularly their race horses.

Lady Cilento did a careful job, took voluminous and detailed notes, and published a thorough report of her findings and conclusions in an Australian weekly magazine called *Woman's Day*. The issue for 12 November 1973 carried the first of three parts of the report. (I know of no comparable weekly magazine in the United States or Canada. The issue to which I have referred consisted of 119 pages, beautifully and liberally illustrated with full-color as well as black-and-white photographs.)

When she left on her tour, Lady Cilento undertook to try to discover the truth about Vitamin E and to report the full story, whether she found the claims for it true or false. In the article she says: " . . . I am convinced that the claims made for alpha-tocopherol are fully justified." She goes on to describe a variety of conditions in which she has seen it work. Finally, she lists in detail seventeen ways in which Vitamin E works in the body.

With her kind permission, I have included part of the 12 November 1973 article as Appendix B of this book. I should like to conclude this chapter now with some excerpts from it that we appreciated very much.

"Whenever I hear people ridiculing the claims of the Shutes," writes Lady Cilento, "calling them 'cranks' and refusing to consider the possibility that Vitamin E may have a saving function in cardiovascular disease, I look again at the list of deaths from heart disease in Australia . . . . I am reminded of the many other occasions when life-saving innovations were delayed for years by the irrational conservatism of the medical Establishment . . . . To the list of [those] men who fought against conservatism and uninformed opinion, history must now add Evan and Wilfrid Shute . . . . Once Vitamin E jumps the barriers of prejudice, it may well be instrumental in saving the lives and sparing the suffering of many thousands . . . who will otherwise die."

REFERENCES

1. Ochsner, A., DeBakey, M.E. and DeCamp, P.J. *Journal of the American Medical Association* 144, 831, 1950.
2. Shute, E.V., and Shute, W.E. *Alpha Tocopherol (Vitamin E) in Cardiovascular Disease.* Toronto: Ryerson, 1954.
3. Shute, E.V. *Your Heart and Vitamin E.* Toronto: Cardiac Society, 1956.
4. Bailey, H. *Vitamin E, Your Key to a Healthy Heart.* New York: Arc, 1964.
5. Shute, W.E. with Taub, H.J. *Vitamin E for Ailing and Healthy Hearts.* New York: Pyramid, 1969.
6. Haeger, K. *Vascular Diseases* 5, 199, 1968.
7. Von Rave, O., Wagner, H., Junge-Hülsing, G. and Hauss, W.H. *Zeitschrift Rheumaforschung* 30, 266, 1971.

7

ALPHA TOCOPHEROL
IN THE BODY

THERE IS AN OLD MAXIM that applies to our critics: "A man convinced against his will is of the same opinion still." Because I believe this to be true, I do not seek to convert our critics. I write now, instead, for interested and intelligent laymen and for doctors who have been in practice long enough to realize that their professors and the officers of their medical associations are not automatically all-knowing because of their exalted positions. I have every expectation that the summary I am about to present of some of the more important research on the treatment of cardiovascular disease in humans with alpha tocopherol will be accepted by such people as logically coherent and scientifically sound.

Since a complete bibliography for this chapter would necessarily be enormous, only a partial one can, for practical reasons, be presented here. (See Chapter 5 for the numbers of supporting papers in each of the main areas.) At the end of the References for this particular chapter, therefore, you will find a special list of nineteen additional readings intended for those who wish to pursue the subject further. These reports will be particularly well worth studying to reinforce the information presented in this chapter.

Let us now think back to the list of functions of alpha tocopherol I gave you in Chapter 5. There was, first, the ability to safely dissolve fresh clots and to prevent their formation. In addition, I listed the ability to reduce the oxygen requirement of the tissues and cells, to decrease abnormal capillary permeability, to function as a capillary vasodilator, to promote collateral circulation and to promote epithelization. I shall now outline for you what we now know about each of these functions.

1. Alpha Tocopherol as an Antithrombin

One of alpha tocopherol's two most important functions is, as we have seen, its ability to dissolve fresh clots and to prevent their formation. (Its ability to dissolve fresh clots is particularly easy to demonstrate in peripheral veins.) In this it is unique both because of its effectiveness and its safety.

Alpha tocopherol is a potent antithrombin and is antithrombic in normal concentration in the bloodstream. As I explained in Chapter 3, this action of alpha tocopherol in its application to human medicine was first noted by our group in 1946. In 1948 a paper by Zierler and his group established that alpha tocopherol is vigorously antithrombic both in vivo and vitro (inside and outside of the living body) and that it is antithrombic in its normal concentration in human blood.

Perhaps the strongest and most persistent advocates of alpha tocopherol as a potent antithrombin are Dr. Alton Ochsner and his group. In 1950 Kay, Hutton, Weiss and Ochsner (2) described the use of 300 IU orally a day in the successful treatment of four cases of thrombophlebitis. In-flammation subsided and edema disappeared. In this same paper they advocated its use along with intravenous calcium gluconate in the prevention of thromboembolic phenomena.

In the same year Ochsner et al. (3) stressed its prophylac-tic use in the *Annals of Surgery*, and Ochsner, DeBakey and DeCamp (4) also pointed this out in the *Journal of the American Medical Association*.

In a letter to the *New England Journal of Medicine* in 1964, Ochsner (5) states that "alpha tocopherol is a potent inhibitor of thrombin that does not produce a hemorrhagic tendency and is therefore, a safe prophylactic agent against venous thrombosis." He reiterated the same conclusions about the value of alpha tocopherol before the fifty-second annual as-sembly of the Interstate Postgraduate Medical Association, and his remarks there were published (6) in *Postgraduate Medicine* in 1968. In the absence of the prophylactic use of alpha tocopherol, there is a steady and frightening increase in thrombophlebitis and pulmonary embolism.

It stands to reason that an antithrombic agent which dissolves fresh clots, which is antithrombic in normal con-centration, and which is effective in preventing intravascular clotting *must* have a role in the treatment and prevention of a whole group of major medical catastrophes. For example, alpha tocopherol is uniquely useful in treating phlebitis, in preventing phlebitis and so preventing thromboembolism, in treating and preventing "strokes," and in preventing the arterial and venous thrombosis complications of Buerger's disease.

2. Alpha Tocopherol as an Antioxidant

Alpha tocopherol's second important function is its abil-ity to decrease the need for oxygen in the tissues and organs of the body. This it shares at megavitamin levels with Vitamin C and with trace levels of selenium. Any two or all three of these can be used together. This action is of great usefulness whenever there is a decreased level of oxygen in tissue. It helps the cells to survive if the reduction is extreme and, in less dangerous situations, to function more normally. It has, therefore, very wide application in many apparently unrelated conditions.

When arteries are narrowed, the availability of oxygen is gradually decreased until it reaches the level at which the cells cannot carry out their normal metabolic functions. If the sclerosing (hardening) process continues, it may reach the point at which the cells can no longer survive and the result may be very serious—gangrene, myocardial infarction or brain softening, for example.

When veins become unable to return blood to the heart at a normal rate, blood which has released a portion of its oxygen in the tissues stagnates there to some degree, and fresh blood and oxygen cannot reach the tissues. In some large varicosities the blood flow can actually be reversed. Edema of the extremities with interstitial fluid prevents the normal transport of oxygen and of the waste products of cell metabolism across the cell membrane.

Whatever the cause, the ability of alpha tocopherol in 300 to 3,200 IU a day to decrease the cell's need for oxygen will help the individual cell and therefore the tissues in general to function more normally or even quite normally. Impending gangrene, cerebral softening or myocardial infarction can thus be prevented. The best evidence that this is so is in cases of intermittent claudication. Happily, the efficacy of alpha tocopherol in this situation is now clear.

We have a large number of photographs of the results of alpha tocopherol treatment in many cases where the deterioration of blood supply, due either to narrowing of arteries or stagnation of blood in the venous system (or both), with or without accompanying intravascular clotting, has led to peripheral gangrene or to ulceration. In diabetic gangrene, the administration of alpha tocopherol helps the cells proximal to the dead cells to regain their normal function, and so to resist extension of the necrosis, and to initiate normal healing processes. Soon an area of demarkation appears and the living tissues literally slough off the dead tissues.

Without alpha tocopherol treatment, such cases inevitably result in amputation of the leg, usually above the knee, since only at this level is the blood supply sufficient to allow the flaps of the stump to heal and eventually, it is hoped, to bear the patient's weight. Many such cases have been allowed to go on to complete self-amputation. The slides we show to medical audiences illustrate this. The results shown in our slides are unique in that no other agent could have saved these legs.

In the heart and brain the same action of alpha tocopherol provides a like result. The eye is an extension of the brain, the latter making up 2 percent of the body weight but demanding 25 percent of the body's total nutrition. The vessels in the retina are readily visible through the dilated pupil since they are covered by a single layer of cells. As a result, all the pathological changes in the arteries, veins and capillaries can be seen and photographed. Hemorrhages, exudates, scars and other types of damage can also be observed. These changes can be reversed by alpha tocopherol. They can be treated even more rapidly and more completely by megavitamin doses of E and C.

Alpha tocopherol is essential for the normal activity of all the cells in the body. Their integrity and function depend on adequate blood supply. When the oxygen supply is reduced by pathological changes in the blood vessels, alpha tocopherol will always decrease the oxygen need and in many cases allow the cells and tissues to behave normally.

Cells can be damaged and their metabolism critically affected by circulating toxins. This occurs in the heart in acute rheumatic fever and in the kidneys in acute glomerulonephritis (a kidney inflammation), and here the action of alpha tocopherol is of maximum value. When given at the onset of symptoms, it allows the heart and the kidney to handle the insult rapidly and completely.

In most pathological lesions for which alpha tocopherol is an adequate answer or is greatly helpful, its antithrombic and antioxidant mechanisms are the ones which lead to the initial improvement as, for example, in the treatment of fresh thrombophlebitis or in the healing of a heretofore intractable chronic ulceration of the leg. However, alpha tocopherol has other important actions which in other cases are the chief reason for its usefulness or the reason for an improvement in rate and degree of recovery.

3. Alpha Tocopherol as a Controller of Abnormal Capillary Permeability

Another most important action of alpha tocopherol is its ability to restore capillary permeability to normal in areas of insult whether allergic or due to infection. It is this action of overcoming the allergic responses and preventing or reversing the damage that is responsible for the rapid and almost miraculous recovery of patients treated at or near the onset of acute nephritis or acute rheumatic fever. This statement should be amended. It is an absolute miracle to see an acute case of either of these conditions return to absolute normal in as little as twenty-four to forty-eight hours. Usually there is every evidence of complete recovery in a matter of days, often in only two or three. The only comparable experience is the witnessing of complete disappearance of all evidence of acute phlebothrombosis.

In a fresh case of acute nephritis or acute rheumatic fever

an infection, usually in the tonsil or throat, triggers a pathological reaction in the kidney in the one instance or the myocardium in the other. The tissues of the organ become waterlogged due to pathological changes in the small vessels and capillaries, and normal metabolism is critically impaired. Alpha tocopherol restores normal capillary permeability. The tissues return to normal and literally throw off the impending damage. Unfortunately, alpha tocopherol is less effective in the chronic stages of these conditions.

4. *Alpha Tocopherol as a Capillary Vasodilator*

Alpha tocopherol also functions as a dilator of capillaries and therefore as a facilitator of the circulation of blood throughout the body. This action is of value in many conditions in which there is spasm in a vessel wall or a significant degree of vessel damage, acute or chronic.

5. *Alpha Tocopherol and Collateral Circulation*

Alpha tocopherol speeds up the collateral circulation in two ways: by reducing any abnormal tendency to spasm and by increasing the size of the collateral channels.

It has been shown experimentally that alpha tocopherol increases the degree of development of collateral circulation and initiates this effect earlier than it would develop otherwise. This network of smaller vessels dilates to carry a larger volume of blood around the block to the vessels beyond. This may provide the necessary help to prevent death of an extremity.

This action of alpha tocopherol is probably the main reason for the observation made early in our experience, and corroborated so often since, that once definite improvement is experienced, it will continue slowly for a long time, usually months, often years. Unlike most treatment, which works to a certain degree and then stops at that level or slowly declines, alpha tocopherol treatment usually continues to bring about improvement in patients. In heart patients this is evidenced not only by their clinical signs and increasing exercise tolerance, but also by the slow but steady improvement, even for years, in their electrocardiograms. The majority of cardiac patients are middle-aged and older. To see them keep on improving as they get older is a most gratifying experience.

6. Alpha Tocopherol and Epithelization

Ulcerated and denuded wounds heal more rapidly with alpha tocopherol therapy, and the scar tissue does not contract and is not tender. For this reason, and because of its ability to limit cell death to those cells that have been killed by the burning agent, alpha tocopherol is the ideal treatment for burns. It will even act favorably on old scar tissue, reducing many scars even to the point of near disappearance. In old keloids, it takes away the itchiness that often accompanies the condition and reduces the redness. Keloids can be prevented by the prophylactic use of oral alpha tocopherol and application of topical (local) alpha tocopherol to the fresh wound. (A keloid is an overproduction of scar tissue in certain individuals. Keloids are more common in the races with heavy skin pigmentation.)

Another action of alpha tocopherol must be mentioned—namely, its general help *by means of all the mechanisms we have discussed* in the treatment of a large group of connective tissue diseases.

The observation by ourselves and others that alpha tocopherol is of great use in many of the collagen diseases (diseases of the main protein constituent of the connective tissues and cartilage) confirms part of the mechanism of the unique characteristics of E-treated lesions. (The German work by von Rave et al. has been cited previously.)

Finally, alpha tocopherol has the ability to combine with other vitamins, minerals and hormones. This was noted many years ago by veterinarians, notably Dr. H.C. Burns of the H.C. Burns Company of California, in the successful treatment and prevention of "white muscle disease" in lambs and calves. Alpha tocopherol was effective but selenium, a trace mineral, more so. Selenium alone, however, is toxic in the effective dose. A small quantity of alpha tocopherol plus the selenium was much more effective than either alone. In addition, the resulting material was nontoxic and 97 percent effective.

There are many such instances. Treatment of hypo-glycemia, for example, is completely successful when three vitamins at the mega level are combined with the appropriate diet. One of these is 800 IU of alpha tocopherol.

In *Executive Fitness Newsletter* for 20 November 1971 there is an account of a study reported at the Fifth Annual Convention on Trace Elements in Environmental Health at the University of Missouri. In this study, Dr. James P. Isaacs of the Johns Hopkins School of Medicine, Baltimore, followed twenty-five heart patients thirty-nine to seventy-five years of age who were classified as "poor risks." Dr. Isaacs gave them a daily dietary supplementation that included Vitamin C (100 mg), Vitamin E (100 IU), a low-dosage vitamin and mineral formula and the trace elements copper, zinc and manganese. Every fourth month, for a month at a time, Vitamin B_6 (100 mg) was also given daily. All but one of these patients was still alive after six years and none of the survivors has had a recurrence of his heart problem or has gone back to the hospital because of heart disease complications. All, including the one patient who died, had experienced improved exercise tolerance. Beneficial side-effects noted were improvement in skin texture and appearance; augmentation of nail pliability, growth rate and cuticle development; improvement in hair density and growth rate and scalp health; and improvement in gum color, texture and healing. It was also noted that "gums and teeth became more strongly attached."

An interesting part of this experiment is the effectiveness of the treatment with only 100 IU of E and 100 mg of C when these were combined with other substances.

The keystone of the research work done by the Shute group and their followers over the years was, as I have mentioned, the interest of my father, Dr. Richard James Shute, in the use of thyroid to neutralize excess estrogen in some of his patients. In 1933 he enthusiastically joined my brother Evan in combining the use of thyroid treatment with Vitamin E treatment.

Estrogen and thyroid extract are antagonistic. Estrogen and alpha tocopherol are also antagonistic. And in people who are low in thyroid activity, cardiovascular damage is increased, both in rate of incidence and in degree. Strangely enough, all this was somehow understood empirically by my father who because of necessity was an industrial surgeon but by inclination was a general practitioner with a special interest in obstetrics and gynecology.

The very real usefulness of E and thyroid (and male sex hormone, which is also an estrogen antagonist) in gynecological and obstetrical problems is the special field of my brother and I shall not, therefore, go into it except in a minor way. But I think it is important here to give you a brief summary of the relationship of Vitamin E, estrogen and thyroid. For one thing, this relationship represents the beginning, in an historical sense, of all of our work. For another, I believe that the relationship itself is an extremely significant one, and one which will continue to unlock many mysteries in medicine in the future, just as it has done for us in the past. For it has led us, I am certain, to what may well be the greatest discovery in medicine in this century.

Let us look, for a moment, at the work of Dr. Paul Starr. He discussed subclinical hypothyroidism in an article in *World Wide Abstracts of General Medicine* (Volume 5) in 1962. This beautifully illustrated article points out that even mild degrees of chronic hypothyroidism, usually not recognized by the patient until he or she has been thoroughly questioned by a knowledgeable physician, lead to increased risk of arteriosclerosis, especially of the brain; myocarditis sufficient to produce heart failure; slow mentation, delayed comprehension, poor memory and loss of initiative; atherosclerosis (hardening of the arteries accompanied by fat deposits in their inner surfaces) with resulting angina pectoris; anemia, resembling either the primary or secondary form; somatic (bodily) muscle weakness, leading to orthopedic disability; anorexia (loss of appetite); constipation, even to the point of obstruction; fibrositis (painful inflammation of fibrous tissue) with body-wide pain resembling gout; and phlebothrombosis, with resulting embolism.

All this is interesting, since the person with hypothyroidism has an excess of estrogen and/or a deficiency of Vitamin E.

Some years ago the *Journal of the American Medical Association* published a leading article entitled, "The Amazing Prevalence of Hypothyroidism in the General Population." It was a report on a statistical study in Chicago of apparently healthy adults. The conclusion was that 55 percent of females (apparently healthy, remember) and 45 percent of males were low in thyroid activity.

It has been suggested that putting iron into bread would help us to deal with widespread anemia in women. Obviously this is not the ideal answer. Putting iron in bread decreases the availability of Vitamin E, and this could well precipitate severe cardiovascular disease—one of the consequences of hypothyroidism listed by Starr. However, correcting hypothyroidism in most of these women would remove the cause of their anemia without reducing the existing Vitamin E supply in their bodies. This would be treating the cause, not the effect.

There is now direct evidence of the dangers resulting from administration of estrogen (or conversely deficiency of thyroid or Vitamin E or both).

Dr. G.T. Mellinger (7) reported in 1967 that estrogen given to males with prostatic cancer significantly increased mortality from cardiovascular disease. This has been confirmed by the Veterans Administration Cooperative Urological Research Group, in an editorial (8) in the *Medical Journal of Australia* and in a letter from Dr. J.C. Bailar (9) in *The Lancet* in 1967.

The administration of estrogens in the birth control pill has many deleterious side-effects, particularly, of course, in those women who are already high in estrogen because they are low in thyroid. In a report to the American College of Physicians, Drs. Weinberger, Collins and Luetscher of the Department of Medicine at Stanford University School of Medicine stated that hypertension developed in patients taking "the pill" after about one year (as high as 215/125 and not below 160/100). Within one to four months after the therapy was stopped, the pressure dropped, and after six months it returned to normal in half the patients. (This was reported in the *Medical Post* for 6 May 1969.)

Estrogen therapy for the inhibition of lactation in women who do not wish to nurse their babies is associated with a threefold increase in the incidence of puerperal (after-childbirth) thromboembolism. In women who have had operative delivery (cesarean section) and who are more than twenty-five years old, the incidence of puerperal thromboembolism is increased tenfold.

The Coronary Drug Project, a national collaborative study to evaluate long-term effects of five drug regimens, including estrogens, reported that the group receiving 50 mg per day of estrogens experienced an excess number of non-fatal myocardial infarctions, pulmonary embolisms and cases of thrombophlebitis, compared with the placebo group. No overall trend in reducing mortality was evident to justify its use, according to the account of this project which appeared in 1970 in the *Journal of the American Medical Association*.

Finally, a report in *M.D. of Canada* in October 1973 on the Boston Collaborative Drug Surveillance Program—a study of a large number of women—revealed that among women taking oral contraceptive pills there was eleven times the incidence of idiopathic thromboembolism and double the incidence of gallbladder disease, when these women were compared with controls.

Low thyroid, high estrogen, low Vitamin E equals a great increase in various cardiovascular lesions!

Physiologically, estrogen compounds cause increased growth of the mammary ducts, with progesterone (another female hormone) stimulating the growth of alveolar tissue (the glands themselves) developed under the influence of estrogen. Patients with chronic cystic mastitis respond to 200 to 400 IU of alpha tocopherol a day for three successive months, according to a report by Dr. A.A. Abrams in the *New England Journal of Medicine* in 1965.

My brother Evan and my younger brother, Dr. Wallace B. Shute, who is also an obstetrician and gynecologist, rarely give their gynecological patients estrogens. Menopausal symptoms in general respond better to alpha tocopherol or to thyroid or to both, and senile vaginitis (inflammation of the vagina in older women) usually responds much better to alpha tocopherol in suppository form. This is not surprising when it is remembered that more than half the women in the general population are already high in estrogen. Since 55 percent are hypothyroid, and many others probably have normal or near-normal thyroid function, there are probably not very many, relatively, who are hyperthyroid and who therefore could possibly benefit from estrogen therapy.

We are not alone in holding this opinion. The *Medical Post* for 20 February 1973 contained a report indicating that the *Medical Letter* had said routine use of estrogens to treat emotional symptoms of menopause has not been shown by "adequate evidence" to be beneficial. The *Medical Letter* also was quoted as stating that estrogens in fixed combinations with male hormones or with vitamins or sedatives have not been proved useful by "acceptable studies . . . for symptoms related to the menopause."

In this brief summary of ways in which alpha tocopherol behaves in the body, I have attempted to sketch for you what some key investigations have revealed. As you can see, not all the evidence is in. The story is not yet complete. We are a lot farther along in our understanding of the various actions of alpha tocopherol, however, than we are in our understanding of the modes of action of some other long-accepted therapeutic agents. The *Medical Post* of 21 March 1972 carried an article on penicillin the first sentence of which is this: "Research workers at the Max Planck Institute in Tibingen, Germany, believe they are on the way to explaining how penicillin works."

Already?

REFERENCES

1. Zierler, K.L., Grob, D. and Lilienthal, J.L. *American Journal of Physiology* 153, 127, 1948.
2. Kay, J.A., Hutton, S.B., Weiss, G.M. and Ochsner, A. *Annals of Surgery* 28, 124, 1950.
3. Ochsner, A., Kay, J.H., DeCamp, P.J., Hutton, S.B. and Bolla, G.A. *Annals of Surgery* 31, 652, 1950.

4. Ochsner, A., DeBakey, M.E. and De Camp, P.J. *Journal of the American Medical Association* 144, 831, 1950.
5. *New England Journal of Medicine* 271, 211, 1964.
6. *Postgraduate Medicine* 44, 91, 1968.
7. Mellinger, G.T. *Canadian Medical Association Journal* 96, 559, 1967.
8. *Medical Journal of Australia* 1, 991, 1971.
9. *The Lancet* 2, 560, 1967.

SUGGESTED ADDITIONAL READINGS
(In chronological order)

Hove, E.L., Hickman, K.C.D. and Harris, P.L. *Archives of Biochemistry* 8, 395, 1945.

Butturini, V. *Giornale di Clinica Medica* (Bologna) 27, 400, 1946. (Electrocardiographic support.)

Lambert, N.H. *Veterinary Record* 27, 355, 1947. (Heart disease in dogs and cats treated successfully. Ruling out the psychological aspect of the treatment of heart disease.)

Pin, L. Thesis. M. Lavergne, Paris, 1947. ("We can confirm the curative properties of alpha tocopherol.")

Zierler, K.L., Folk, B.P., Evzaguirre, C., Jarcho, L.W., Grob, D. and Lilienthal, J.L. *Annals of the New York Academy of Sciences* 52, 180, 1949.

Dedichan, J. *Nordisk Medicin* 41, 324, 1949. (Patients definitely benefited on Shute dosage.)

Galeone, A. and Minelli, M. *Minerva Medica* 46, 694, 1950. ("Electrocardiographic regression particularly significant.")

Schmidt, L. *Medical World* 72, 296, 1950. (Fifty-one cases with satisfying response.)

O'Connor, V.T. *Medical World* 72, 299, 1950. (Good results in sixty cases.)

Enria, G. and Ferrero, R. *Archivio per le Scienze Mediche* 91, 23, 1951. (Marked and rapid development of collaterals around occluded vessels. Complements the preceding paper and explains continuing improvement over a long period in alpha tocopherol-treated patients.)

Crump, W.E. and Heiskell, E.F. *Texas State Journal of Medicine* 48, 11, 1952.

Telford, I.R., Wiswell, O.B., Smith, E.L., Clark, T.R., Jr., Tomashefski, J.F. and Cricuolo, D. Air University School of Aviation Medicine, Project No. 21-1201-0013, Report No. 4, May 4, 1954 (Randolph Field, Texas).

Puento-Dominguez, J.L. and Dominguez, R. *Revista Espanola de Cardiologia* 9, 30, 1955. (Induced infarcts in canine hearts with arteriographic evidence of increased vascularization in the ischemic areas due to alpha tocopherol.)

Diaz, F.V. *Progresos de Patol y Clinica* 3,351, 1956. (The use of alpha tocopherol is of indisputable value in treating coronary disease.)

Harman, D. *The Lancet* 2, 1116, 1957. (Interesting comment on use of highly unsaturated fats and consequent increase in body's need for Vitamin E. These fats also inhibit enzyme action. Author on staff of Veterans Administration Hospital, San Francisco.)

Livingston, P.D. and Jones, C. *The Lancet* 2, 602, 1958. (One of the significant double-blind studies on peripheral vascular disease. Recommends at least three months' trial.)

Sautter, H. *Deutsche Medizinische Wochenschrift* 83, 1514, 1958. (Reversed retinal arteriosclerosis and other eye pathologies with Vitamins A and E.)

Jacques, W.H. *Canadian Medical Association Journal* 81, 129, 1959. (Eight hundred to sixteen hundred units of alpha tocopherol used in chronic polio patients with peripheral vascular lesions, with relief of symptoms in three to four weeks. Symptoms recurred if alpha tocopherol discontinued.)

Kawahara, H. *Surgery* 46, 768, 1959. (Alpha tocopherol used in venous thrombosis. Sixty-seven percent successful.)

8

HEART ATTACKS: CAUSES, SURVIVAL AND PREVENTION

FOUR THOUSAND of the world's leading cardiologists assembled recently in England at the Sixth World Congress of Cardiologists. There was much discussion of myocardial infarction and an "awareness" that it was "probably becoming more common"—rather an understatement, in my opinion, since its incidence has now, as we have seen, reached epidemic proportions. Disappointingly, the Congress yielded no new suggestions concerning effective treatment or prevention of this condition.

Considering the high incidence and the seriousness of myocardial infarction, there is surprisingly little in the usual treatments for it that is, in my assessment, of very much use to its victims. And again, considering the incidence and the seriousness, there is also surprisingly little concerning its underlying causes that is understood with complete certainty.

Until very recently, for example, it seemed to be universally believed that in cases of myocardial infarction the proximate cause was a thrombus or, occasionally, some other kind of obstruction, in a branch of the coronary artery which blocks it off. It was accepted that the tissues of an area of myocardium, thus deprived of their essential blood supply, died, were absorbed and were replaced with scar tissue. It is now believed by some, however, that an infarction may in some cases *precede* development of the thrombus. In such cases the immediate cause of myocardial infarction would not be coronary thrombosis but *acute myocardial hypoxia* (deficiency of oxygen in the affected tissues of the heart).

How often this may happen is disputed. A 1971 editorial in the *Canadian Medical Association Journal* states that it may happen more often than some in the field have thought. And Drs. D.M. Spain and V.A. Bradess (1) have suggested in the journal *Circulation* that thrombosis is so often found at autopsy simply because the patient survived long enough after the infarction for thrombosis to develop in the coronary artery.

It has, strangely enough, been found that narrowing to the point of complete occlusion of the coronary artery can occur *without* necessarily causing infarction. According to a paper by Dr. G. Baroldi (2) in the *American Journal of Cardiology*, this is because of well-developed anastomotic (communication) pathways around areas of coronary stenosis (narrowing) which have almost always been present when such cases have been examined. What is even more interesting is the converse—the idea that there is some mechanism in the heart muscle that can lead to its death independent of coronary thrombosis. This is intriguing because it fits in with some other interesting observations indicating that deficiency in certain natural antioxidants (Vitamins E and C) whose job it is to protect dietary unsaturated fatty acids may be at the root of this deadly mechanism.

Such a deficiency state has actually been found, both in animals and in men, by Dr. T.W. Anderson in cooperation with Malcolm D. Wilson, a pathologist, Anthony A. van Dreumel of the Veterinary Services Laboratory, Ontario Ministry of Agriculture and Food, and Richard E.C. Hutson of the Toronto East General Hospital. A paper on this in *The Lancet* (3) states that a singular correlation has been found between the microscopic lesions in the animal disease, nutritional muscular dystrophy, produced when dietary unsaturated fatty acids are inadequately protected by antioxidants, and the lesions found in middle-aged men who had died suddenly of acute myocardial infarction. According to *The Lancet* for 20 October 1973, the animal and human lesions were morphologically (structurally) indistinguishable.

I shall make reference later in some detail to work by Dr. H. Glatzel, who has shown that the incidence of myocardial infarction rose abruptly between 1951 and 1953 when the public became convinced that the use of polyunsaturated fats would protect against coronary disease or the recurrence of myocardial infarction after recovery from the initial attack. For the moment, just think of what this may mean in the population that is deprived of much of its dietary Vitamin E. Remember also what Dr. Tappel had to say on the same subject. He pointed out that Vitamin E was needed to protect unsaturated fats and noted that people who consume large quantities of polyunsaturated fats need an especially high E intake, even after giving up such a diet.

Recently there has been support for—but not complete acceptance of—this new concept of myocardial infarction: that it will, at times, occur *prior* to the appearance of a thrombus. Dr. A.A. Tambe and his group (4) in a 1972 issue of the *American Heart Journal* have offered some new evidence in support of this concept, whereas in the same year a paper by Dr. D. Sinapius (5) a German pathologist, in *Deutsche*

Medizinische Wochenschrift reinforces the older idea of "a temporal and causal sequence of coronary artery thrombosis and myocardial infarction."

Whatever the mechanism of the occurrence of myocardial infarction, the incidence of such attacks is steadily rising. Some patients have symptoms of coronary insufficiency or an embarrassed myocardium before the acute attack, in the form of vague precordial distress (discomfort in the heart region) often associated with eating or exertion. A fair proportion of these have been to their doctors. In the absence of electrocardiographic changes, most of these patients have not had their real problem diagnosed. However, only a minority of men who have an initial myocardial infarction—even a rapidly fatal episode—have had these earlier signs such as angina, hypertension, congestive failure, other cardiovascular disease or diabetes.

The percentages of immediate, early and late deaths from myocardial infarction vary so widely from report to report in the journals that it is difficult to give accurate survival figures. You will remember, for example, that I have quoted Dr. Bernard Lown of Boston as saying that 65 percent of infarction cases in the United States never reach the hospital or are dead on arrival. By contrast, Dr. Charles W. Frank (6) of the Albert Einstein College of Medicine stated in the *Bulletin of the New York Academy of Medicine* in 1968 that the initial attack is fatal in one-third of cases. Of all deaths, more than 85 percent occurred on the first day.

Dr. G.E. Dimond (7) stated in 1961 that in a group of patients surviving one to two months after the initial attack, there was a 55 to 66 percent chance of living five years, and that 50 percent of second and 92 percent of third infarctions were fatal. A 1968 paper by Dr. Eve Weinblatt and associates (8) stated that 36 percent died in less than one month after the initial attack. The probability of surviving 4½ years after the initial infarction was 52 percent (compared to Dimond's 55 to 66 percent). The risk of a first recurrence was still high (4½ years after the initial infarction) in comparison with the risk of a first infarction in the general population, underlining the ongoing effect of first myocardial infarction in later prognosis.

In other words, the factors that allowed the patient to have a first attack were still present, unaffected by any measure suggested as treatment or prevention by his physician. He remains at great risk.

The extent of the damage to the heart muscle in the initial attack, and consequently the chance of survival (or, if the patient lives, the degree of disablement) depends on many factors. Site of the occlusion and its rapidity are important. Then again, no two hearts have the same blood supply. Although the coronary arteries follow a general pattern in all hearts, there are many variations within this. Some people are born with an unusually good coronary tree. Some, however, have relatively poor or unevenly developed coronary blood supply, and some have inadequate vessels in one or two areas. Others are well endowed with collaterals—those smaller vessels which by their connections at different levels can carry blood around occluded or narrowed major vessels.

Similarly, the degree of arteriosclerosis in the rest of the blood vessels and the condition of nutrition in the rest of the heart are factors in survival. The resistance of the individual to the initial shock is still another factor, and the presence of other pathological conditions such as hypertension, valvular disease, lung disease or diabetes also has a bearing. All of these things may have an effect on the patient's survival and on the degree to which he recovers if he does survive.

There is variation in this aspect of the reports, just as there is in the survival statistics in the various studies. For example, in Dimond's group the presence of hypertension was associated with a poorer prognosis but the effect of over-weight was not statistically significant.

Something else that I consider very interesting is often stated as an afterthought in such papers. Frank, for example, adds that "serum cholesterol concentration did not relate to prognosis in the 2½-year period after baseline examination. Men with values exceeding 260 mg percent did not have significantly higher infarction or death rates than those with values less than 220 mg percent."

Dr. Berthold Kern, one of Germany's leading heart specialists, claims that obesity, a high cholesterol blood count and excessive cigarette smoking are not important causes of heart disease. (But he suggests that excessive agitation and aggravation and too little rest may be the important causes. That is interesting since Sir Maurice Cassidy, the King's physician, long ago, stated that in his lengthy experience, stress did not appear to be a major factor in coronary disease!)

Differences of opinion, to the point of confusion, pervade almost every aspect of the field of cardiology. And in virtually all aspects of this field, the "authorities" have been in gross error. Their inability to get results is a matter of record. Let me illustrate.

At a meeting in Baden-Baden, Germany, of the International Society for Combating Heart Disease, Dr. Kern said that in his opinion the forty billion dollars expended over the past forty years in research into the causes of heart disease had produced no really proved and practical results.

And Dr. W. Stanley Hartroft, former Research Director of the Hospital for Sick Children in Toronto, has said: "Heart disease has us beat." No progress, he said, had been made in fighting heart disease. He went on to note that doctors hand out advice on how to minimize the chances of heart disease—stop smoking, eat less animal fat, lose weight—yet have no proof that these measures are effective.

Finally, Ancel Keys, Ph.D., the man chiefly responsible for the nearly world-wide acceptance of the role of ingested animal fats, came to a meeting of the Second International Symposium on Atherosclerosis in Chicago in 1970, and had this to say: " . . . nothing has been altered in the slightest" by a quarter century of intensive work. "Despite systematic studies of the epidemiology of heart disease, there have been no advances whatever in the basic goal of prevention."

The mention of Dr. Keys, who is Director of Minnesota's Laboratory of Physiologic Hygiene, brings me to the story of cholesterol. It is just impossible to assess the damage done by the anti-cholesterol theory. The amazing part of the history of this is the almost instant acceptance of the cholesterol idea as soon as it was promulgated by Keys, its effect on the treatment of thousands of patients restricted uselessly and unnecessarily in their diets, as well as on the dairy, poultry and meat-processing industries. All of this was to no avail. At one time, he even had airlines interested in sending in blood samples from their pilots. Yet all this money and effort produced no results of any value, by his own admission.

Time magazine for 30 June 1967 reported the curious situation of the chairman of the AMA Executive Committee on Diet and Heart Disease. This was during the height of the Keys-inspired interest in cholesterol. *Time* said that in light of the many deaths of men under seventy from coronary artery disease, there had been considerable interest among doctors in establishing whether changes in diet could help. Could enough men be persuaded to try a low-fat diet and stay with it?

"At last week's A.M.A. meeting, the Executive Committee on Diet and Heart Disease reported after a long-term pilot project involving 2,000 men aged 45 to 54 that it was indeed possible. The next step, said the committee, is to seek more conclusive proof by enlisting up to 100,000 men aged 40-59 in a new $50 million study."

Forty thousand men on a low-cholesterol diet were to be compared with forty thousand other men for at least eight years! At a cost of fifty million dollars! A fascinating sidelight was the condition of the chairman, Dr. Irvine H. Page, aged sixty-six, who did not attend. Said *Time:* "Though he has kept slim, exercised often and followed his own low-fat regimen for years, he was recovering in Cleveland Clinic Hospital from a mild heart attack." More significant still was the good doctor's explanation of his heart attack. It wasn't the cholesterol, it was his "drive and competitiveness"—not even stress or overwork. Perhaps in other cases it also has not been dietary fat.

This brings us, naturally, to the American Heart Association which each year begs (and obtains) millions for heart research. It also puts out a booklet entitled *Reduce Your Risk of Heart Attack* whose preface states that "in the midst of the greatest abundance this country has ever known, Americans are faced with a baffling health problem." This booklet has these suggestions to make—and I shall make some comments on them very shortly:

1. Reduce the saturated fat and cholesterol in the diet.
2. Reduce your weight if you are overweight.
3. Control high blood pressure.
4. Exercise.
5. Eliminate cigarette smoking.
6. Control diabetes.

Finally, the pamphlet suggests that a family history of heart attacks in middle age may be of interest to the man who wants to prevent one in himself. How, I wonder, is he to change his parentage? Also, how many heart attacks could there be among a man's ancestors, since there *were* no heart attacks prior to 1912 and very few prior to 1930?

As to the Heart Association's suggestions, I can agree completely only with Number 3. It is true that since the introduction of potent anti-hypertensive drugs the death rate from hypertensive heart disease has decreased by 50 percent. However, this is an area in cardiology in which the failure to *use* successful therapeutic agents is all too common. (This will be discussed in Chapter 11.)

As to number 2, I can only say that overweight has no relationship to heart disease directly. Reducing your weight, if you are overweight, can only help you indirectly, by reducing the many miles of extra vessels supplying the excess fat in the obese body, and therefore reducing the heart's work to some degree.

There is an obvious and definite connection between obesity and overeating in many cases, and this apparently begins in childhood with excessive consumption of starchy foods and sweetened products. (So many foods now contain refined sugar—a substance which has no nutritive value, just empty calories.) However, there is a much more important relationship—that between hypothyroidism and obesity. Most hypothyroids are obese—mostly because they do not burn up energy normally. And as pointed out so clearly by Paul Starr, hypothyroidism is associated with an increased incidence of cardiovascular diseases and anemia. This important relationship has been so universally missed or ignored by the profession in general.

Simply expressed, obesity is often due to hypothyroidism and this is why it is associated with an increased incidence of cardiovascular disease. It is not obesity that increases the danger of heart attacks: it is the condition that leads to the obesity that is the culprit. Reduction in weight thus has really very little effect in reducing the danger of cardiovascular disease.

A recent confirmation of this was published in *The Lancet* by Dr. P.A. Bastenie et al. (9) and Dr. R. Calay et al. (10), who showed that preclinical (asymptomatic) hypothyroidism is not uncommon and that this condition increases significantly (by 2½ times) the risk of coronary artery disease in women.

As to Number 4 (exercise), I have many doubts. So far, it has been shown only that exercise, if indulged in sensibly and in moderation, does no harm to the person who has not yet had a myocardial infarction. It has not been shown to be useful to the patient who has had an infarction. It has initiated many fatalities among the latter and may well precipitate an attack a little earlier than would otherwise have occurred in some people.

Following nationwide reports in Sunday magazine supplements of happy members of a coronary club jogging around an indoor track at the Cleveland Y.M.C.A., a similar program was initiated at the Y.M.H.A. in North York, a suburb of Toronto. Newspapers carried pictures of that cheerful group jogging along. The only trouble was that the instructor supervising their jogging and participating with them dropped dead of a heart attack!

The Scientific Advisory Committee on Atherosclerosis of the Ontario Heart Foundation has issued a warning to the public and the medical profession to the effect that "physical training should always be initiated as a gradually increasing program of activity. . . . This is an individual problem, particularly in persons with known heart disease, in which case gradual, limited exercise *may be beneficial or may be very harmful.*"

The warning continues: "Generalizations that exercise is good or bad for patients with heart disease (or any other disease) are not possible and such patients should always consult their own physician about their problem."

The Committee's statement goes on to say it is not known whether life is prolonged by exercise. Daily exercise "within the limits of one's ability" is approved, however, for healthy people and for "medically 'selected' patients with heart disease." Selection criteria, which the Committee says "should be used cautiously," were listed as follows:

1. More than three months post infarct.
2. No heart failure.
3. No heart enlargement radiologically.
4. No angina at rest.
5. No recent increase in severity and frequency of exertional angina.
6. No prolonged angina on effort which is not relieved in a few minutes by rest.
7. Stable EKG pattern.
8. No serious arrhythmias at rest or after exertion. Patients with single infrequent ventricular ectopic beats or with paroxysmal atrial tachycardia (rapid heart beat of sudden onset) may be admitted to the program if the arrhythmia is not precipitated or aggravated by exercise. (Definition mine.)

Obviously, these criteria define a person with nearly complete recovery from an attack—a nearly normal person —the exception. I repeat then: the value of exercise in preventing attacks of coronary occlusion has not been established.

Cigarette smoking (Number 5) is often said to be a factor, but universal agreement on this is lacking. Remember, Dr. Berthold Kern, the German specialist, gave it as his opinion that excessive cigarette smoking was not a factor! I believe, however, that it is certainly an undesirable habit, one that can do no one any good—and one which by constricting peripheral blood vessels, could be mildly harmful.

As to Number 6, the control of diabetes, I must agree that this is undoubtedly worthwhile in preventing deaths from diabetic coma or insulin reactions. But the usual methods of controlling diabetes apparently do not prevent the rapid, almost universal cardiovascular changes that are characteristic of this disease and thus are not a factor in preventing heart attacks.

As to Number 1, the comment about cholesterol, it may be worthwhile to point out that numerous experts have disagreed with the proponents of this idea ever since it was first put forward—but with very little effect.

As early as 1960 Dr. Howard Sprague, a former president of the American Heart Association, told the annual meeting of the Canadian Heart Association to ignore the cholesterol fad. He reminded his audience that cholesterol is synthesized in every body tissue except the brain. In 1962 Dr. Philip L. White, Secretary of the American Medical Association's Council on Foods, released to United Press International an official warning which was printed in nearly every newspaper on the North American continent. This was a statement calling the "anticholesterol fad" a wasted effort that could be dangerous. In *The Lancet* for 11 September 1965, the Research Committee announced that there was no significant reduction in mortality rate following the use of a low-fat diet in proven coronary artery disease. And in 1970 Drs. Shanoff, Little and Csima stated in the *Canadian Medical Association Journal* that neither the level of serum cholesterol nor that of the lipoprotein fractions (substances containing fats and proteins) is related to survival. (Anyone who is interested in further information on this should read the comments of Dr. Meyer Texon of New York in the 31 May 1971 issue of the *Journal of the American Medical Association.*)

Another useful article on the cholesterol controversy is

one by Dr. E.R. Pinkney in *Medical Counterpoint* (1971). A condensation of this appears in an issue of *The Summary* and also in Appendix C of this book.

In the condensation there is the comment that although serum cholesterol level "has become the principal indicator of the health of one's heart and blood vessels to both public and . . . medical profession," we still do not know from "good clinical evidence that a diet-lowered serum cholesterol in any way prevents or modifies heart attacks or heart disease."

It also points out that serum cholesterol is hard to measure because any stress, even a small one, can alter it. There is also the statement that serum cholesterol level only drops 3 for each 100 mg removed from the diet and that it has not been shown that as a result of reduction of serum cholesterol levels the cholesterol actually leaves the body!

In addition, the condensation points out that there is "ample evidence that heating polyunsaturates tends to resaturate (or polymerize) the product and so defeats the very purpose for which polyunsaturates are promoted. Resaturation of the polyunsaturates by heating occurs in family cooking." If, as so often happens, cooking oil is reused, "the degree of saturation becomes even worse."

And let me quote here some other paragraphs from the same condensation that I think are particularly interesting:

> Heating an unsaturated oil (especially corn oil) to 200° for 15 minutes (far less than normal cooking temperatures and time) actually enhances atherosclerosis in animals.

> In Kumerow's study all his animals on a diet containing heated corn oil developed tumors, and only one of 96 survived the 40 month experimental period. None of the animals fed only fresh corn oil developed tumors; all survived.

Men on a high P.U.F.A. [polyunsaturated fatty acids] diet showed a 65 percent greater incidence of cancer than controls on a standard diet. The J.A.M.A. [Journal of the American Medical Association] reporting this finding also noted that those on the high P.U.F.A. diet also had 70 fatal atherosclerotic accidents as compared to only 48 such deaths in the controls; a similar ratio was found for myocardial and cerebral infarcts.

Polyunsaturates may be a primary source of the radicals inside the cell that cause aging.

Recently the *Canadian Medical Association Journal* carried a report from overseas which highlighted a controversy over "risk factors" conducted in the columns of *Medisch Contact*, a Dutch publication. In March, 1974 *Medisch Contact* printed an article in which it was maintained that "large-scale screening and intervention in respect of risk factors for heart and vascular disorders" was not justified. In the opinion of the authors, such factors were not yet defined with sufficient clarity. The authors also stated, according to the *Journal*, that "there was so far no evidence that manipulating the risk factors would prevent coronary disease." On 24 May 1974, the same Dutch publication carried rejoinders.

I find this exchange interesting because it illustrates the fact that many people in a number of countries now doubt the entrenched "cholesterol approach" to the prevention of coronary disease.

Even more significant is a United Press International report *(Palm Beach Post* 23 January 1975) concerning the results of a five-year governmental trial of five different cholesterol-reducing drugs. More than eight thousand coronary patients were studied in the hope that the drugs would prove effective in reducing death rates and cutting the incidence of recurrent heart attacks.

According to the UPI account, "three drug treatments were dropped early in the trial because they were doing more harm than good." The remaining ones, according to the same account, "proved to be of no benefit when results of groups taking the drugs were compared with a group taking a dummy drug."

I am not surprised, of course, that this elaborate test by professional researchers has failed to demonstrate that use of these cholesterol reducers prevents recurrences. But I am wondering when researchers are going to give up completely on this line of inquiry. The director of the project was quoted as saying that the results applied only to older persons already having had heart attacks and not to primary prevention, and also that diet might still be helpful in lowering high cholesterol levels.

However, the final assessment of the value of the American Heart Association's help for the person interested in preventing heart disease is perhaps most effectively made by borrowing some words once more from my favorite cardiologist, Dr. Eliot Corday. Commenting in the 1973 interview with a medical writer in the *Los Angeles Times* to which I have already referred, Dr. Corday noted that although for quite a few years many patients have been "avoiding risk factors," this has not caused the death rate from coronary artery disease to decline. "Let's tell our patients," said Dr. Corday, "that we believe this advice should be followed but that we have no real proof that eliminating the risk factors will prevent progression of the disease."

Fortunately for the thousands of heart patients we have been able to help over the years, there is, and has been for some time, a better approach. And there are, of course, two aspects to this: first, treatment of heart attacks and prevention of recurrences, and second, prevention of initial attacks.

As Dr. A. Ernest Mills first pointed out in a letter to me in

1947, the myocardial infarct patient given an adequate intake
of Vitamin E immediately will develop the characteristic
changes in the electrocardiogram, but to a diminished degree
and with a more rapid and more complete return to normal
than the patient who survives his attack without E.

Emergency treatment should include intravenous and
oral coronary dilators for the obvious reasons that any increase in coronary blood flow through the unobstructed portions of the coronary circulation and the dilatation of any
collateral circulation present could minimize the area of
anoxic myocardium and thus the extent of immediate shock.
The relatively minor help so obtained may allow the patient to
survive who might otherwise not do so. A further hope is that
dilatation of the vessel involved in the thrombus before it
becomes attached to the wall may allow the blood proximal to
the clot to push it further into the artery and possibly break it
up. That this does happen in peripheral arteries has often
been demonstrated. In the case of myocardial infarction without preceeding thrombosis of the artery, vasodilation may
also be helpful in flooding the anoxic muscle with an increased volume of blood.

The patient should be put to rest in bed in a sitting
position since the heart works more efficiently in this position, and given morphine to decrease pain and "allay apprehension." As soon as he is pain-free, he should be allowed
up in an armchair with care that the seat is so arranged that
the pressure on his thighs is evenly distributed and that the
front of the cushion does not dig into the back of the thighs.
As soon as he can swallow, he should be started on 1,600 IU of
dl-alpha tocopherol and given at least that quantity daily.
Bathroom privileges should be allowed from the beginning.
When patients are so treated, the mortality rate will be under
10 percent.

After the first ten days the patient should be ambulatory.

He should be ready for discharge by the end of the third week. Judging by recent reports, it may even be safe to increase activity after the second week, and many patients can return to work six weeks after the infarction.

The main reason that used to be given for the six weeks of absolute bed rest—the prevention of aneurysm of the ventricular wall—does not apply, apparently, since the incidence of this is not increased by Levine's armchair treatment. It may actually be diminished since the myocardium is probably better nourished when the patient is allowed to sit up.

When the patient has had hypertension, the fall in blood pressure that occurs with the infarction makes it perfectly safe to use a full dosage schedule of alpha tocopherol. After recovery, the pressure usually does not rise again. If it does rise, it is rarely as high as its original level and can be treated as soon as it becomes necessary with the modern antihypertensive drugs.

In the patient with normal blood pressure before the infarction, and whose pressure has inevitably dropped, the ability of alpha tocopherol to improve the tone of heart muscle can greatly help to speed up the return of pressure toward a normal range.

After discharge from the hospital, continuation of the same level of alpha tocopherol is usually all that is needed. Occasionally it will be obvious, then or at a later date, that a particular patient may well benefit still more from an increased level of dosage.

There is the general observation, made by all those familiar with alpha tocopherol therapy for myocardial infarction —and our experience is huge over the course of twenty-five years—that the patient who has had an infarction and has survived is almost fully protected from any later attack.

So much for treating heart attacks and preventing recurrences. But what are the chances of avoiding an attack in the first place?

The evidence that alpha tocopherol is prophylactic depends upon two observations. First, there is the definite proof first shown by Ochsner's group and confirmed many times since, that in the case of venous thrombosis not only can the fresh clot be lysed (dissolved) but further episodes prevented. Ochsner and his associates have also shown, of course, that alpha tocopherol used prophylactically in a large series of surgical cases will decrease the incidence of venous clotting and, according to Ochsner, absolutely prevent the occurrence of pulmonary embolism. The second is the observation to which I have just referred—namely, that with alpha tocopherol therapy the patient who has had a myocardial infarction and survived is almost fully protected from recurrence.

There is, of course, direct proof of the prophylactic value in preventing coronary thrombosis in myocardial infarction in the papers of Boyd and Haeger. Both showed that there was a definite decrease in deaths in their series of patients being treated for intermittent claudication.

By deduction, then, it is probable that the majority, though not all, who would take 800 IU of alpha tocopherol daily and faithfully would escape a myocardial infarction. This is probably true of all those who have blood pressures in the normal range and who have not had rheumatic fever. (The subject of how much alpha tocopherol can safely be given to persons with high blood pressure or chronic rheumatic heart disease—and under what circumstances—will be discussed in Chapters 9, 13 and 16.)

It would seem, however, in the light of increasing knowledge of the action of other vitamins, chelated minerals and thyroid hormone and of the deleterious effects of our increasingly polluted environment, the processing of our foods, the removal of essential nutrients from them and the addition to them of so many chemical substances, that the expectation of prevention would be greatly enhanced by correction of these complicating factors.

REFERENCES

1. Spain, D.M. and Bradess, V.A. *Circulation* 22, 816, 1960.
2. Baroldi, G. *American Journal of Cardiology* 16, 859, 1965.
3. Anderson, T.W. *The Lancet* 2, 298, 1973.
4. Tambe, A.A., Demany, M.A., Zimmerman, H.A. and Mascarenhas, E. *American Heart Journal*, 84, 66, 1972.
5. Sinapius, D. *Deutsche Medizinische Wochenschrift* 97, 433, 1972.
6. Frank, C.W. *Bulletin of the New York Academy of Medicine* 44, 900, 1968.
7. Dimond, G.E. *Circulation* 23, 881, 1961.
8. Weinblatt, E., Shapiro, S., Sager, R.J. and Frank, C.W. *American Journal of Public Health* 58, 1329, 1968.
9. Bastenie, P.A., Vanhaelst, L., Bonnyns, M., Neve, P. and Staquet, M. *The Lancet* 1, 203, 1971.
10. Calay, R., Kocheleff, P., Jonniaux, G., Sohet, L. and Bastenie, P.A. *The Lancet* 1, 205, 1971.

9

ANGINA AND RHEUMATIC HEART DISEASE

TO HEAR MOST PEOPLE TALK—and to skim the mass media—one would often think that the only kind of heart disease is the "heart attack." Certainly the occurrence of a myocardial infarction possesses a kind of stark drama—often, indeed, tragedy—and that is undoubtedly part of the reason, along with its ever-mounting incidence, that it receives so much public attention. It is all too easy, therefore, for most people to fail to grasp the plight of the four to five million men and women who suffer from angina pectoris and the 1.6 million victims of rheumatic heart disease.

The term *angina pectoris*, as I have said, simply means pain in the chest. But of course a pain is a symptom, not a disease, and there are many underlying conditions which can produce such a symptom. The disease state known as angina pectoris, however, is a definite one with a definite cause:

myocardial anoxia. The pain is referred from a heart muscle that is temporarily deficient in oxygenation. The deficiency may be in a small area of the heart or it may be a generalized deficiency.

Like coronary thrombosis, angina pectoris is a condition that has developed relatively recently in the long history of man. Dr. Michaeles, writing in the *British Heart Journal* in 1966, pointed out that Medieval and Renaissance physicians in England and Wales have left no description of a pain resembling it. He mentions a 1768 description of angina by Heberden, an English physician, but comments that the condition seems to have been very rare then and even later.

In 1973 the *Medical Post* carried a quotation from a book by Dr. Austin Flint which was published in 1866 and entitled *A Treatise on the Principles and Practices of Medicine*. Dr. Flint describes angina as a rare complaint, and he substantiates this statement by saying that there were only seven such cases in more than a hundred and fifty instances of organic heart disease that he had studied, and none at all in the cases of cardiac disease he had seen in the five years preceding the time at which he wrote.

According to Michaeles, Sir William Osler (1849-1919), the great physician who described several cardiovascular diseases, saw no cases of angina pectoris in twelve years of clinical work.

Just how serious is this condition that gets so little public attention and that is of such relatively recent genesis? What is the outlook for patients with angina pectoris?

Dr. William B. Kannel reported to the twentieth annual meeting of the American College of Cardiology that one in four men and one in eight women with angina pectoris can expect to have a coronary attack within five years. Thirty percent of those over age fifty-five will die within five years.

Forty-four percent of the coronary deaths will be sudden. Abnormal electrocardiograms (EKGs) are ominous signs in angina pectoris: less than 50 percent of patients with such EKGs survive five years. Survival in men with uncomplicated angina pectoris is no better than in those with angina pectoris following in the wake of myocardial infarction.

Many different treatments have been known to relieve pain of angina pectoris.

All doctors use nitroglycerine for relief of angina. Nitroglycerine, either under the tongue or orally, does reduce the length of the anginal attack in most cases, although an inert pill is often as effective. In spite of the widespread use of nitroglycerine and of the good results ascribed to it, there have been many papers which have denied its effectiveness. (When longer-acting but similar compounds are used, some patients report a definite decrease in the number of episodes.)

Dr. Russek, to whom I referred in Chapter 2, has treated 102 patients suffering from severe angina for six years with a combination of drugs—one which slows down the heart and reduces its need for oxygen, and one which dilates the blood vessels and increases blood flow to the heart muscle (without, however, altering the basic pathology). His patients experienced about the same mortality rate from heart attacks as is expected among apparently healthy people in the same age range.

A succession of operative procedures has been developed, each of which was at first said to yield 75 percent success with very low mortality. Unfortunately, it is hard to make a firm evaluation of these since angina has a trick of responding to placebos, both pharmaceutical and surgical.

A sham operation in which the skin is incised under anesthesia and sewn up again will often relieve angina. And according to Dr. Eliot Corday, the 60 to 90 percent relief reported by proponents of the coronary bypass operation must be compared with the 60 to 70 percent success of the sham operation.

As Corday also points out, these surgical claims must also be compared with the 60 percent success reported by users of placebo pills (inert pills having no known therapeutic value).

A further difficulty is that the placebo pill used to make comparisons with the results of surgery or nitroglycerine or other forms of treatment is not really inert. It has been shown by extensive research that placebos, by affecting the autonomic nervous system, can cause many different symptoms such as coughs, pain, headaches and vomiting—and angina pectoris itself! It seems, therefore, that other methods of clinical investigation may be preferable.

It is our position that treatment for angina pectoris must include alpha tocopherol, for independently of whether or not it abolishes or even diminishes the symptoms it must increase the chances for survival. Alpha tocopherol, in fact, should and usually will abolish the symptoms, or at least greatly reduce the frequency and severity. In patients who develop angina following upon a myocardial infarction—a common situation in such recovery periods—the angina is usually relieved in from four to six weeks after initiation of treatment with alpha tocopherol.

Acute rheumatic fever is a heart condition whose incidence is decreasing owing to the introduction of the sulfonamides and the antibiotics. Adequate, immediate treatment of streptococcal infections in the upper respiratory tract will prevent acute rheumatic fever. However, when the acute stage develops ten days to three weeks after tonsillitis or pharyngitis of other inflammation in this area, the antibiotics are of no value. Neither is anything else, except Vitamin E. Salicylates, cortisone and other drugs that are sometimes tried only treat symptoms and do not prevent the progression to heart damage and chronicity.

The incidence of acute rheumatic fever could be greatly lowered if all streptococcal infections were adequately treated with antibiotics. However, acute rheumatic fever is often so mild that it is undiagnosed. It is also extremely difficult to make a firm diagnosis of rheumatic heart damage in the asymptomatic stage. When surgeons first found that they could open the human heart, they found that cardiologists' diagnoses were "not often wrong but usually wrong," to put it in words I have heard used by a prominent Canadian heart surgeon. Often it is only when a man or woman reports for an insurance examination or for one requested by an employer who has been sold on routine annual physicals that a lesion is picked up. Almost half of those who have rheumatic heart disease give no history of an acute episode and cannot believe that they have any heart lesion.

Where acute rheumatic fever does develop, its seriousness could be much reduced if it were treated adequately and immediately with alpha tocopherol. A difficulty, however, is the fact that such treatment must be prolonged. It is very difficult to persuade a good many patients with proven rheumatic lesions who are nevertheless asymptomatic to follow a course of treatment with alpha tocopherol which is expensive and which must be carried out daily, faithfully and continuously.

There is no more dramatic proof of the therapeutic action of alpha tocopherol than its effect on acute rheumatic fever. All signs and symptoms disappear in as little as forty-eight hours after treatment is begun. The only other comparable examples are in the treatment of acute nephritis and acute thrombophlebitis.

With any other treatment, however, a large percentage in all three of those conditions go on to chronicity. In the case of rheumatic fever, the proportion is about 80 percent. Many of these patients have recurrences of the acute phase, but the majority make an apparently complete recovery and have years of apparently normal health while the connective tissue lesions characteristic of the disease are continuing to develop and progress. Ultimately, valvular lesions start to produce symptoms. The chronic rheumatic heart patient is to be pitied, since once his symptoms develop the disease progresses slowly but inexorably and the patient becomes a chronic invalid.

Much can be done for these chronic cases. Obviously, however, the time to treat them is in the very early acute stages when the disease can be eradicated, the heart protected and chronicity prevented.

The first symptoms of chronic rheumatic heart disease are usually shortness of breath or a pounding of the heart on exertion or excitement, a little more than usually experienced previously. Then a little typical unproductive cough begins, followed by a little orthopnea (discomfort that occurs whenever the patient tries to breathe unless he is sitting straight up or standing up). These patients respond beautifully to alpha tocopherol treatment, so well, in fact, that I have treated many without seeing them.

For example, while on vacation in Florida some years ago, I received a telephone call from a friend in New York who wanted to see me at once. I knew that he had had rheumatic fever in childhood and that a mitral lesion had been found some years previously. Now he had developed serious early symptoms of mitral stenosis (narrowing of the opening of the mitral valve) and had just been investigated in the heart section of a university hospital. After cardiac catheterization (a diagnostic procedure in which a tube is passed into the heart through a vein or artery) he was told that he had a severe degree of mitral stenosis and that he would need an immediate operation. They actually booked him for this operation. It was then that he called me.

I asked his symptoms and then asked if he was still working. He said he was.

"Every day?"

"Yes," he replied.

I told him he didn't need surgery and that he would be as well as he had been ten years before if he would take Vitamin E correctly. Here is where the right dosage schedule of a properly assayed and labelled product is absolutely crucial. The dosage is absolutely precise, 75 IU a day for a month with no obvious benefit, then 100 IU a day for a month with no obvious benefit, then 150 IU a day and a virtual guarantee that six weeks after beginning 150 IU he would be free of symptoms.

This is exactly what happened in this case (and in nearly all others of this type). Alpha tocopherol is almost 100 percent effective. My friend now lives a normal life. On the one occasion on which I have seen him since—a social one—he was completely asymptomatic and had been dancing all evening the night before. He now works on the third floor of a building and for sheer exhilaration takes the two flights of stairs two steps at a time!

There was something that my friend had not told me previously. This was that during his catheterization he had suffered a cardiac arrest. In spite of this he submitted, when he was called back to the hospital for a checkup eighteen months later, to another cardiac catheterization and once more suffered a cardiac arrest. He knew the dangers involved but by now was so interested in the clinical improvement in his condition that he wanted to know if there was definite evidence of this that would be revealed by catheterization. After this second catheterization he was told that he had mitral stenosis and that *some day* he would need corrective surgery. When he asked why he was originally an emergency but not any longer, no explanation of his excellent clinical status was forthcoming. (Of course the diagnostic murmur of mitral stenosis will always be present to some degree.)

Unlike patients with early symptoms of chronic rheumatic heart disease, rheumatic heart disease patients who have developed serious heart failure—and particularly those with auricular fibrillation (fast, irregular heartbeat)—are very difficult to manage. These patients need all the treatment of their complications that can be devised as well as the alpha tocopherol on the 75-100-150 IU regimen. If they are fibrillating, but not otherwise, they must have the dosage of a digitalis preparation that will regulate their apex heart rate (the rate obtained with a stethoscope at the apex of the heart). They may also need diuretics in the amount necessary to drop them to a basic weight and keep them there.

Such patients will usually show very worthwhile improvement and if they do, improvement will continue for many months. But they need frequent re-evaluations, particularly of their dosage levels of diuretics and digitalis. Most who initially need diuretics can reduce or eliminate them after four to six months of treatment, but it should be stressed that these patients respond slowly—a characteristic of Vitamin E treatment mentioned often before in relation to this condition and others, particularly intermittent claudication, as we shall see in Chapter 11.

It is now more than two hundred years since William Withering wrote his treatise on the value of the foxglove in treating dropsy. Since that time, volumes have been written on the proper use of digitalis, yet it is one of the most misused and abused drugs in the pharmacopeia.

The *Medical Post* for 12 December 1972 carried an article that states that 33 to 50 percent of patients on digitalis are not being optimally managed. This is alarming after two hundred years! There is such a narrow margin between therapeutic and toxic effects. It is mentioned in this *Medical Post* article that Dr. Thomas W. Smith of Harvard has stated that of 900 consecutive admissions to the Harvard Medical Service emergency ward, 135 were digitalized prior to admission and that among these the incidence of definite digitalis toxicity was 32 percent. An additional 6 percent had possible digitalis toxicity.

The same article says that Dr. Roger W. Jelliffe, Associate Professor of Medicine at the University of Southern California School of Medicine, has reported the incidence of adverse reactions at 20 to 30 percent of hospitalized patients. Dr. Jelliffe's team recently studied ninety patients who had been receiving digitalis by the conventional method and whose digitalis dosage subsequently was computed by a new computer-assisted method. Thirty-five percent of the patients had adverse reactions to the drug when their doctors used the conventional method.

The use of digitalis and Vitamin E by the same patient requires constant surveillance. Vitamin E usually reduces the dosage level of digitalis needed by these patients, and the usual maintenance level used by most physicians is often too much, sometimes much too much. It must be remembered that digitalis is a highly selective poison—very useful and very dangerous. Today it has only one function of importance: the regulation of the apex rate in the patient with auricular fibrillation. There are so many more potent and safer diuretics that its usefulness as a diuretic can be ignored, and the general statement that digitalis increases the output of blood from the heart may well not be of much importance here. Digitalis should be given to the chronic rheumatic heart patient who is fibrillating—not otherwise.

Digitalis intoxication is commonly seen in patients in our practice, especially when the family doctor insists on chang-

ing our routines. Since diuretics as well as Vitamin E poten-
tiate the action of digitalis, the latter is just too dangerous a
drug and wholly unnecessary except in the fibrillator.

A second—and also very important—point that must be
made concerning the use of Vitamin E in chronic rheumatic
heart disease is that dosage and schedule, as I have already
said, must be handled with the utmost care and precision.
Giving a chronic rheumatic heart disease patient 300 IU a day
will lead to tremendous improvement in some cases within
three to seven days. *However, it will make many more such
patients much worse, and that rapidly. If continued, it will kill them.*
Only in the rare case when the damage to the two sides of the
heart is equal will the patient be able to tolerate and benefit
from 300 IU a day. Since, in most cases, one side of the heart is
more severely damaged than the other, even 300 IU will help
the better side faster than the more damaged side and will
thus throw the heart into worse imbalance. Incipient heart
failure can be precipitated or, if there is already failure, it will
be rapidly increased. *Thus, the correct 75-100-150 IU schedule is
of the utmost importance.* The patient should be told that no
improvement can be expected until he or she has been on 150
IU for four to six weeks.

All other precautions in the use of alpha tocopherol are
also of special importance in these cases. Inorganic iron neutralizes alpha tocopherol if the two meet in the gastrointestinal
tract. Iron in medicine form cannot be given, therefore, with
Vitamin E. Since the blood level of Vitamin E is maintained
much better when it is given in divided doses at least twice a
day, this is the way it should be used. When iron must be
given, the Vitamin E must all be given at one time and all the
iron eight to twelve hours later. It should also be remembered
that mineral oil absorbs Vitamin E and does not readily release
it, whereas vegetable oils do release it readily. Mineral oil
should be avoided. Another important consideration is the

fact that estrogens are Vitamin E antagonists and, since dosage is crucial in these cases, estrogen should be avoided.

Very few patients are allergic to Vitamin E preparations.* When they are, one of the other forms can usually be used without a reaction. There are three forms: the so-called natural, its succinic acid salt, and the synthetic.

Although I have not had a long and therefore adequate experience in the simultaneous use of megadoses of ascorbic acid (3 to 5 gm or more a day), I have reason to suspect that Vitamin C should be used with caution in treating chronic rheumatic heart disease. Vitamin C apparently reinforces the action of E since C is a water-soluble antioxidant, and the 150 IU of Vitamin E, along with C, may therefore produce effects resembling those of using larger amounts of E.

It is curious that the chronic rheumatic cases respond to only 150 IU of E a day and that this may be the maximum needed. Nevertheless, we always try to give as much as 300 IU eventually, reaching that level only after months at a lower dosage. By contrast, coronary and—as we shall see in the next few chapters—peripheral vascular—cases need much more before full response is obtained—somewhere in excess of 800 IU a day and often as much as 2,400 to 3,200 IU a day.

---

*However, see Chapter 15 for discussion of some allergic reactions to the ointment.

10

ATHEROSCLEROSIS AND AN
IMPORTANT BREAKTHROUGH

IT MAY WELL BE PREMATURE to announce now, in this book, another most important medical discovery. But I think that this new advance is so vital to the health of millions of people that I cannot resist giving you at least some background and basic information about it. It suggests a valuable adjunctive therapy to alpha tocopherol treatment and a universal use in the prophylaxis of the aging process in blood vessels.

As is so often the case with major discoveries, this one came about as a result of the more or less chance meeting of minds and pooling of knowledge of a small group of investigators—in this case, Dr. Frederick Klenner of Reidsville, North Carolina, Dr. Morgan Raiford of Atlanta and myself. And this is only one of the worthwhile consequences of the formation of an organization known as the International Academy of Preventive Medicine five years ago by a small group of doctors.

The objective of the Academy is to provide a platform for clinical investigators, biochemists and researchers in all sections of the healing arts who are interested in preventing degenerative diseases as well as in providing alternatives to acute disaster crisis medicine. Its activities include the organization of meetings twice a year which are open to all who are interested in the field of preventive medicine so that they may meet and hear the leaders in their field and participate with them in question-and-answer panel discussions. The organization has grown numerically beyond the fondest dreams of the organizers: it now has more than five hundred members. Speakers of the highest caliber have presented their works at these meetings and each meeting seems to surpass the previous ones.

At the meeting in Detroit in October 1972, a magnificent presentation on the action and clinical use of massive doses of ascorbic acid, orally and intravenously, was given by Dr. Klenner. The next day, just before I was to present my paper on the actions of alpha tocopherol, he came up to me, introduced himself and said, "If you want another testimonial, here's one." He handed me a four-by-five-inch piece of paper on which was written:

> Since Sept. 1, 1970 I have been taking 5000 to 6000 d-alpha tocopherol along with 20 gm. Vit. C. At that time, I had classical heart failure being sensitive to Inderal (a drug that slows the heart and reduces its oxygen need). After two years, my heart is back to normal in size and EKG. (Definition of Inderal mine.)

I asked him how much enlarged his heart had become

and he said, "Maximum." He added that he had a whole series of x-rays showing its steady enlargement and its return to normal size, and that the large intake of Vitamin C did not help his condition until he added the very large daily amount of d-alpha tocopherol.

This was too good a result for Vitamin E alone, and so this complete recovery must have been due to both together. It has been established that Vitamin E protects Vitamin A and that Vitamin E also undergoes other important nutritional interactions, including interactions with the trace element selenium and the sulfur amino acids methionine and cysteine-cystine.

Dr. Klenner's experience was most significant. Here was a clinical application of the interaction of Vitamin E and Vitamin C. Dr. John Barker, who has taken over my practice in Mississauga, Ontario, Canada, and I immediately began to apply this information to all our coronary and hypertensive heart disease patients as well as to our cases of peripheral vascular disease. Certainly they have done well.

Now for the interesting sequel, but first a basic explanation.

Following the experimentation on dogs by the medical student Floyd Skelton under the direction of my brother Evan, our small group began to treat cardiac disease chiefly and a few peripheral vascular cases as well. We submitted our results to a meeting of a medical society and presented papers to medical journals. In our innocence, although we knew of the vicissitudes of other innovators in the medical world, we expected the interest of physicians and especially of cardiologists.

Instead, we became involved in medical politics to a degree we had never dreamed possible. Even the disappearance of massive anasarca (spreading of fluids into connective tissue) and peripheral edema in our first three cases was ascribed by one cardiologist at the meeting of the Ontario College of Physicians and Surgeons to the forceful personality of the doctors treating these patients. This was a particularly interesting statement since one of these patients—the one with the most extreme fluid retention—had originally been his. Obviously he didn't have a forceful personality!

Because of the opposition to our observations and reports on these cardiac patients and because of the life-saving qualities of the drug, we decided to fight the battle in the field of peripheral vascular disease, where results were measurable and visible. We decided, that is, not to engage in extensive studies on conditions like angina pectoris where placebos have often produced very good results and where even the diagnosis can be more difficult given the variety of conditions which can engender pain.

We decided, at any rate, to go ahead in peripheral vascular disease. We treated ulcers on the legs whether due to arterial or venous insufficiency or both. We treated diabetics who, because of the changes in their arteries due to their disease, had developed gangrene of toes or heels. We treated cases of Buerger's disease, burns, osteomyelitis with draining sores and ulcers, and trauma that denuded large areas of the body, after multiple surgical grafting had failed.

Slides of these my brother and I have shown to many meetings—meetings of doctors and laymen alike. They have never failed to convince viewers of the unique value of alpha tocopherol. What viewers did with their knowledge was a matter for their consciences. Suffice it to say that as a result of our work and our publications, there are many, many physicians throughout the world using it just as we do and, of course, with the same results. It is impossible to know how many there are, since they obviously do not need to communicate with us. Details of our treatment have been published and distributed widely, however, and there are many confirmations through a few other reliable channels such as distributors of Vitamin E preparations and some of the professionals we have met at medical conventions.

The point here is that these slides of peripheral vascular cases demonstrate the effect of massive doses of alpha tocopherol, and alpha tocopherol alone, on tissues with reduced blood supply. Vitamin E is an oil-soluble antioxidant, Vitamin C is a water-soluble antioxidant, and it is known that they complement each other. However—and this is most important—although Vitamin E has been shown to slow down or even halt the progress of atherosclerosis (hardening of the arteries, with deposits of fat on their inner surfaces), it does not always do so. Professor Boyd of the University of Manchester did tell Dr. Yousuf I. Misirlioglu of Switzerland that he observed decalcification (the opposite of hardening) of arteries in some of his patients due to the Vitamin E treatment of intermittent claudication. But now there is *absolute proof* that arteriosclerosis can be reversed and prevented.

This is a most significant medical discovery, and it will not only save countless lives, but make healthful living more common and longer lives more enjoyable. The work was done by Dr. Raiford, an ophthalmologist who is Director of the Atlanta Eye Clinic and Hospital in Atlanta, Georgia.

The problem of atherosclerosis has been the subject of much research. It has been suggested that if arteriosclerosis could be prevented life could be greatly prolonged. In the words of Dr. S. Sherry (1): "Thrombosis has become the prime health hazard of the adult population of the Western World." The answer, at least in part, to thrombosis has been known since 1946. Now it is to be hoped that the answer, at least in part, to atherosclerosis has been discovered. It is also to be hoped that the members of "the Establishment" will behave like scientists and develop its tremendous potential for the good of all mankind.

The importance of arteriosclerosis can hardly be understated. The *Medical Tribune* for 12 July 1972 reported that severe coronary artery disease had been demonstrated angiographically (by means of radiographic study of the blood vessels) by Navy cardiologists in young asymptomatic, physically active men who volunteered to undergo cardiac catheterization because of a family history of coronary artery heart disease and hyperlipemia (an oversupply of fats in the blood). Approximately one in every two subjects, all under age forty and all performing the routine physical duties of Navy fliers or Marines, had "severe, diffuse coronary artery disease involving two or more vessels, with 50 percent or more occlusion." This was reported to the American Medical Association meeting in San Francisco.

According to Dr. J.N. Morris (2), writing in *The Lancet* in 1951, there had been no increase in the prevalence of coronary atherosclerosis in autopsy material at the London Hospital between 1907 (at which time there was no coronary thrombosis) and 1949 (at which time coronary thrombosis was nearing its epidemic status). But the years 1945 to 1953 presented an even more interesting picture.

At the Las Vegas meeting referred to earlier, Dr. Hans Nieper showed a most interesting slide. He kindly had sent to me the source paper in *Arztliche Praxis* for November 1971 from which this slide was taken. The author was Professor Dr. H. Glatzel, to whom I referred briefly in Chapter 8, but the graph was after that of Bansi and co-workers.

The illustration shows the relationship between coronary artery sclerosis and myocardial infarction for the years 1945 to 1953, revealing that there was no real increase in the incidence of the sclerosis during this time. Actually, it had dropped in all but three of these years, yet the incidence of myocardial infarction rose (from very little in 1945) at a steady rate until an important change took place. This was the gen-

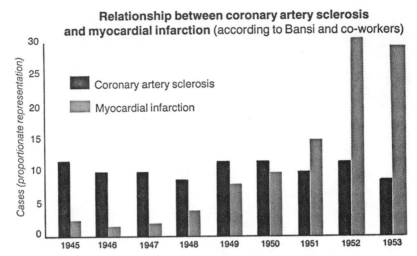

Relationship between coronary artery sclerosis and myocardial infarction (according to Bansi and co-workers)

eral acceptance by doctors of the suggestion that the fat in the diet should be changed to the polyunsaturated type, as in cooking oils and margarines, and that there should be a reduction in saturated fats in the diet. At this stage, the incidence of myocardial infarction rose abruptly, with the 1952 and 1953 figures being in the range of twelve times the 1945 statistics and the 1952 rate three times that of 1950!

This graph was extended to the year 1973 by Dr. Nieper and shown at the March 1974 meeting of the International Academy of Preventive Medicine. The incidence of myocardial infarction had continued to increase while the degree of coronary arteriosclerosis remained essentially unchanged.

This graph illustrates what we have always known and have stated many times, that there is no causal relationship between coronary arteriosclerosis and myocardial infarction. Dr. Glatzel mentioned this in the article from which the graph was taken, pointing out that there was no relationship between the degree of coronary artery atherosclerosis and the clinical symptoms of coronary heart disease. There can be a very severe degree of atherosclerosis in humans who remain free of clinical symptoms. And conversely, there are cases of death with the diagnosis of coronary insufficiency and, at autopsy, the finding of nearly clear coronary arteries!

In Chapter 1 you will find this statement: "The third thought I want to plant firmly in your mind at the outset is this. Up to the time this is being written, cardiologists have, for some strange reason, virtually always done everything wrong and never yet done anything right . . . . " This graph illustrates this by providing one more example. This is one more tragedy that has occurred as a direct result of the inevitable acceptance by cardiologists and, through them, by the majority of physicians, of the wrong concepts.

And it is just amazing that the American Heart Association is totally unaware of this situation and continues to promote this tragic recommendation concerning polyunsaturated fats, and that the American College of Cardiology does the same. Not only that, but they have been, on occasion, willing to lend their official support to a company which manufactures a margarine which contains saturated and polyunsaturated fats, the latter in excessive amounts.

In regard to the recent evidence concerning the action of Vitamin E and Vitamin C in reversing atherosclerotic lesions—and I shall describe it for you very shortly—an interesting article appeared in the *Medical Post* of 8 February 1972. It referred to the British pathologist Dr. Constance Spittle who, in an article in *The Lancet* for 11 December 1971, had suggested that "atherosclerosis is a long-term deficiency of Vitamin C which permits cholesterol to build up in the arterial system." She believes that cholesterol is mobilized from the arterial wall itself.

Back to the work of Dr. Morgan Raiford. The retina of the eye, as I have said earlier in this book, offers an unique area for the direct observation of blood vessels. Since the arteries and arterioles, veins and venules there are covered only with a thin transparent layer of tissue, one can see all anatomical details very clearly. As a consequence, pathological changes in the vessels can be clearly demonstrated. And now, with modern equipment, these changes can be photographed in color or in black and white.

Dr. Raiford's contribution to medical knowledge is his visual proof that the arteriosclerotic lesions in the vessels of the retina due to hypertension, to the aging process or to lesions characteristic of diabetes mellitus can actually be reversed by Vitamin E and Vitamin C, used together in doses of 1,200 IU of Vitamin E and 3 to 5 gm of Vitamin C.

Vitamin E favorably affects the results of blood vessel narrowing, as does Vitamin C to some degree. Both, together, reverse the basic pathology.

Also, the condition known as xanthomatosis, in which there is a visible deposit of yellow-colored xanthoma cells in the eyelids, can be reversed and the deposits in them removed by the combination of Vitamins E and C. Until this discovery, surgical removal of the deposits was the only available treatment.

There have been three previously published methods of combating arteriosclerosis, and very definite evidence that they have been successful. They should be described in detail.

There are now several centers in the United States at which intravenous chelation (a process by which calcium trapped in the walls of blood vessels is removed) is being done by means of a synthetic amino acid whose name is *e*thylene*d*iamine *t*etra *a*cetic acid. It is universally referred to, of course, as EDTA.

The calcium disodium and disodium salts of this acid are very commonly used in a variety of foods to remove trace amounts of metal contamination which might be dangerous and which, in addition, impair the taste, odor or appearance of food, cause beverages to become cloudy, fruits and vegetables to become discolored and fats to spoil. Combined with

BHT and propyl gallate the EDTA salts help prevent oxidation.

EDTA is used in many salad dressings, margarines, mayonnaises and sandwich spreads to prevent rancidity. It is also used in processed fruits and vegetables such as potatoes, peas, corn and mushrooms to prevent browning and in fruit juices to protect Vitamin C against oxidation. Other foods and beverages in which EDTA is used are canned shellfish, beer and soft drinks.

This useful acid should be used very carefully in all these foods because if more than is necessary to trap the contaminating metals in them is used, it will trap also the calcium and other useful nutrients and prevent their utilization by the body.

The medical use of EDTA preceded its industrial use. Because of its unique ability to trap metal ions, it has been used intravenously to treat acute metal poisoning. It is safe because the body rejects it along with the trapped metal ions which are then excreted in the urine. As a result, another growing epidemic—lead and other heavy metal poisoning from contamination of the air by the automobile and by chemical plants—can be treated.

The ability of EDTA to trap calcium in the walls of blood vessels and remove it has led to two other important uses —the treatment of some forms of arthritis and of arteriosclerosis which has reached the stage of calcium deposition in plaques. Removing the calcium by this process (intravenous chelation) leads, apparently, to a breakdown of the soft material in the plaque. My personal experience with this process has confirmed its value in treating peripheral arteriosclerosis and in restoring circulation to critically deprived legs and arms and to cerebral vessels.

The drawbacks of intravenous chelation are obvious. It requires extended treatment in hospital or in outpatient clinics or in specially equipped doctors' offices where considerable extra space is needed. A further drawback is that careful chemical control is necessary, since the process depletes the body of some necessary factors which must be returned in adequate amounts by appropriate oral supplements. Its rapid acceptance, chiefly through the basic work of Doctors Carlos Lamar of Miami, Florida; Dr. Ray Evers, now of New Orleans, Louisiana; Dr. H. Rudolph Alsleben of Anaheim, California; and Dr. Hans Nieper of Germany, is the best measure of its success in the cardiovascular field. Properly used, it is a safe procedure.

Very recently their successes have become known to a much larger group of physicians who have formed the American Academy of Medical Preventics and who have proceeded to pool their knowledge and learn as much as possible before equipping their offices with the expensive but necessary equipment for proper pre-treatment evaluation of the patient. (Each of the members of the AAMP has now added intravenous chelation to his treatment schedule.)

An extensive review of the pertinent literature, a detailed exposition of the clinical uses and method of administration, and the precautions that must be observed is available from Paul H. Huff, 1506 Longview Drive, Fullerton, California, 92631. To those physicians who read this book and are interested in this technique, I can recommend this man as being one whose knowledge is profound and as a source of information.

Another method of preventing and reversing already established arteriosclerosis was developed by Yousuf I. Misirlioglu, M.D., B.Sc., D. Med. Sc. (Basle), M.Sc. (Surg.), F.R.C.S. (C), F.A.C.A., F.I.C.A., F.I.C.S. (I give his degrees in full since they compel careful consideration of his concept!)

The full report was printed as the leading article in the *Summary* for December 1967, and the evidence is certainly convincing. The patients treated were mainly in the advanced stages since they all showed evidence of calcification in the media of the arteries.

Treatment consisted of 400 mg of mixed tocopherols (so-called natural Vitamin E), 400 mg of pyridoxine (Vitamin B6) daily before lunch and 100 mg of nicotinic acid (Vitamin B3) three times daily after meals, increasing to 300 mg three times daily, if tolerated. In addition, he eliminated certain foodstuffs and encouraged exercise—all this to increase fibrinolysis (chemical dissolution of fibrin, a coagulated protein).

Results were obtained in three to six months. X-rays demonstrated complete decalcification of vessels. The foodstuffs prohibited were those containing cholesterol plus coffee, beer, wine, cider and cigarettes. Gin, whiskey, vodka and tea were not prohibited. His work has also been published in *The Lancet* (3) and in the *Medical Tribune* in 1963.

Dr. Hans Nieper has published an account of successful reversal of arteriosclerosis by the use of various salts of orotic acid.

There have been other successful and, incidentally, pretty well ignored methods of treatment designed to lessen the conditions arising from the gradual, progressive narrowing of arteries. The work of the Vascular Research Foundation deserves mention here. For the last forty years this group, of which Dr. Murray Israel is the Medical Director, has had success in reversing diabetic retinopathy and other arteriosclerotic lesions by the use of thyroid and megavitamin B components.

Another investigator interested in this field is Dr. Broda O. Barnes of Fort Collins, Colorado. He has produced quite definite evidence that thyroid deficiency plays an important role in the genesis of atherosclerosis and that thyroid therapy is effective in reducing morbidity and mortality in diabetes mellitus. The role of thyroid deficiency in the development of hypertension has also been investigated by Dr. Barnes. It is interesting, thus, to see my father's work on one aspect of hypothyroidism and its interrelationship with alpha tocopherol, Dr. Paul Starr's work, the work of Drs. Klenner, Israel and Barnes and that of the Shute brothers all leading to progressively greater understanding and control of and ability to reverse arteriosclerosis.

A letter I received in February 1973, and which is reprinted in part below, shows how much was accomplished in one case, apparently by means of alpha tocopherol alone.

Twice in the early part of 1972 I had two very severe attacks of nausea, dizzyness which lasted approximately an hour after which I fell asleep and woke without any ill effects. But played it safe and stayed in bed the next day.

My doctor was unable to diagnose my illness and could offer no remedy against its re-occurrence.

I am 76 years old—have had a slight heart condition for about ten years but nothing serious. I am retired.

Talking to a friend who is an M.D. (but is not accessable as he does not live near me) and telling him of these two attacks, he suggested that I might take Vitamin E pills—400 IU a day—as he had had results which were good with patients who he thought might not be getting enough blood in their brains and Vitamin E supposedly helped keep the proper veins and arteries open in the neck allowing a sufficient supply of blood to reach the brain.

This I have done for the past five months and have had no more of these night attacks.

Have you had such cases and do you find the

supply of blood reaching the brain has been helped by taking 400 IU of Vitamin E daily?

Isn't it curious that the only suggestions for combating arteriosclerosis should involve vitamins, orotic acid salts and a synthetic amino acid? Truly, orthomolecular, megavitamin treatment appears to be the most important new discovery and promises to initiate an era of medicine—an era in which the ravages of civilization and aging can be somewhat ameliorated.

Anyone interested in intravenous chelation will find that there is a new textbook in this field by H. Rudolph Alsleben, M.D. and Wilfrid E. Shute, M.D. entitled *How to Survive the New Health Catastrophes*. It was published in 1972 by Survival Publications Inc., 710 Euclid Avenue, Anaheim, California 92801.

REFERENCES

1. Sherry, S. *Annals of Internal Medicine* 69, 415, 1968
2. Morris, J.S. *The Lancet* 1, 69, 1951.
3. Misirlioglu, Y. *The Lancet* 2, 496, 1966.

11

INTERMITTENT CLAUDICATION

ARTERIOSCLEROSIS CAN AFFECT vessels in any area of the body—the vessels supplying the brain, heart, kidney, other organs or extremities. It can be a very spotty disease, with one area of a vessel showing gross changes while neighboring areas are quite normal. However, this condition when well advanced usually affects several important areas, often well removed from one another.

Arteriosclerotic changes in the vessels of the legs commonly accompany serious changes in the coronary vessels supplying the heart. Often associated with these is a serious involvement of the vessels of the neck supplying blood to the brain. It is well to understand the gravity of the situation once the vessels to the legs have shown a sufficient degree of atherosclerosis to cause the beginning of the cramping pain in the muscles of the calves that is called intermittent claudication.

Drs. T.B. Begg and R.L. Richards (1) of the Western Infirmary, Glasgow, have reported on 198 cases of uncomplicated intermittent claudication followed for five to twelve years or to death. The overall mortality was 46.5 percent; the mortality at five years was 25 percent. Most of the deaths were due to cardiovascular disease, with myocardial infarction as the most common lesion.

Begg and Richards also described further aspects of this condition. Neither age nor the duration of the disease affected the prognosis, nor did the level of the occlusion or whether it was unilateral or bilateral. Elevated blood pressure or coexisting arteriosclerotic heart disease was more important.

The overall amputation rate was 7.1 percent. Most significant was the comparison of the ten-year survival rate of patients with intermittent claudication and those patients who had recovered from a myocardial infarction, or who had angina pectoris. The death rate for those with intermittent claudication was approximately the same as the latter group—those with angina and those who had recovered from an infarction.

Dr. W.B. Kannel and associates (2) have written that as a result of the Framingham study they concluded that there were twice as many deaths from cardiovascular disease when the patient had intermittent claudication as when he had no peripheral vascular symptoms.

Another study of the prognosis of chronic arterial occlusion of the lower extremities was published by Drs. R.W. Hacker and R. Decker (3) in 1968. They analysed the results in 769 patients (703 men) over an eleven-year period.

In the Hacker and Decker group, average age of onset was 51.6 years in men, 63.9 in women. Two stages are described. In Stage One, the complaints were pain induced by prolonged fixation in one position, easy fatigability and parasthesia (feelings such as numbness or burning). In Stage Two there was pain on walking.

Diabetes mellitus was the most important pre-existing disease, and 97.9 percent of the men were smokers. Coronary insufficiency was present in 40 percent of those who had survived to age seventy; gangrene developed in 49.1 percent. During the eleven years 29.5 percent of the group died. The causes of death were cardiac failure, circulatory failure, myocardial infarction and cerebrovascular accidents.

Treatment for this disease has been varied. Vasodilators have been universally prescribed, but there is now ample evidence that they have no real value. (This has been confirmed by Haeger's series.) Anticoagulants and lipolytics (substances causing the chemical decomposition of fats) are of little value, and surgical removal of arterial obstruction has seemed, in the opinion of some surgeons, the best approach. Yet, according to Dr. Robert L. Richards' textbook on peripheral arterial disease, only 10 percent of patients with intermittent claudication require or benefit from surgical procedures. And Drs K. A. Myers and W.T. Irvine (4) reported in 1966 that lumbar sympathectomy (removal of all or part of a nerve in the lumbar region) did nothing to increase blood flow or to improve clinical response in the vast majority of patients.

When the patient has come to amputation the mortality rates are "grim," according to Drs. M.G. Otteman and L.H. Stahlgren (5). Their series consisted of 323 patients with an average age of sixty-seven. Three-fourths of them had cardiorespiratory disease and one-third were diabetics. Gangrene was present in 82 percent and serious local infection in one-third. One-third of these patients required amputation of both legs. The overall mortality was 39 percent with 10 percent dying of unrelated conditions more than thirty days after surgery. It could be that the enforced bed care of those with bilateral amputations hastened their deaths, since this may well be responsible for the onset of bronchopneumonia. Cardiorespiratory disease doubles the risk; the presence of diabetes did not increase it.

In 241 of the 323—nearly three-quarters of the patients—significant complications arose: stump infections, pneumonia, pulmonary emboli or myocardial infarctions. Consider these grim statistics when looking at the proven benefits of alpha tocopherol therapy.

We now believe that there should be a combination of three procedures.

By far the most important of these—and the one now most completely confirmed—is the use of adequate quantities of an adequate preparation of alpha tocopherol. It must be remembered that there are now at least thirty-five papers in the medical literature confirming the excellent response of this condition to alpha tocopherol.

Perhaps the first besides ourselves to present definite data on a large series was Dr. A.M. Boyd, Professor of Surgery at the University of Manchester, and his group (6, 7), who published their findings in 1949. In 1958 Drs. P.D. Livingstone and C. Jones (8) reported a double-blind controlled series in Sheffield, England. One group of patients was given 600 IU of alpha tocopherol a day for forty weeks, the other a placebo with an identical appearance. To avoid bias, the key to the test was not opened until all the results had been declared. Out of seventeen patients who were found to be in the alpha tocopherol-treated group, thirteen had significantly improved, as opposed to two of the control group of seventeen. Six months later none of the improved patients on Vitamin E had deteriorated, and improvement was reported by three controls given Vitamin E after the initial trial had terminated.

It is to be noted—as we have insisted from the beginning—that there is great individuality in the dosage of alpha tocopherol necessary to obtain a response. A double-blind study such as this uses an average dose, adequate for the majority but probably not for all. Further, as these authors and the Boyd group have emphasized, large doses are necessary over a considerable period, at least three months, before satisfactory response is obtained. Boyd added one further important observation: that the E-treated patients had an increased survival. Obviously, the alpha tocopherol also helped the cardiac conditions associated with claudication in many instances, and preserved and prolonged life. He also noticed decalcification of the arteries in a few cases. These comments appear in a later Boyd paper (9) published in 1963. By this time his series of treated patients numbered 1,476 plus another 33 who were used in a blind controlled trial of alpha tocopherol.

The most recent series of papers is that of Dr. Knüt Haeger and his group in Sweden. Dr. Haeger has contrasted the number of amputations in a group of patients treated with other medications against the number in a group treated with alpha tocopherol in a trial lasting quite a few years. I have referred to this study previously. The ratio was 11:1 in favor of alpha tocopherol.

In this study thirty-seven patients were treated with vasodilators and forty-four others with an anticoagulant. Forty-four more were treated for "a period long enough to permit conclusions of the value of [this] treatment" with a multivitamin preparation, and then were switched to alpha tocopherol. In addition, 104 patients were treated from the beginning with alpha tocopherol, initially 600 IU, later 300 IU.

The length of time individual patients were treated varied. The "minimum time of observation" (except for subjects who were switched from the multivitamin to the alpha tocopherol) was two years. In 69.2 percent of cases the period was longer than three years, however. Nineteen of the non-tocopherol group died, compared with nine of the tocopherol group. Moreover, the alpha tocopherol group and the remaining patients showed other differences which Haeger classified as significant. Nearly four times as many on alpha tocopherol increased their walking distances and ten times as many of these more than doubled the distance they could walk without experiencing pain. Particularly noticeable was the amputation situation. The development of intractable pain and/or gangrene caused amputation of twelve legs, only one of which was in the original alpha tocopherol-treated group—again, a significant difference.

In intermittent claudication, we have another example of a condition in which there has been no effective treatment until the advent of alpha tocopherol therapy, but which now yields to this therapy supplemented by megavitamin ascorbic acid and exercise. (The patient suffering from intermittent claudication is very hard to motivate to take regular daily walking exercises. He must walk daily as energetically as possible for an hour, resting when the pain becomes too great. In a treadmill study by Drs. O.A. Larsen and N.A. Lassen (11) reported in 1966, the walking distances increased by as much as three times after six months of exercise. Four of these patients improved to the point at which they could walk normally on the flat for as long as they wished without pain.)

The rationale for the effectiveness of alpha tocopherol therapy in intermittent claudication remains the same as for its usefulness in other cardiovascular pathology—a decrease in oxygen need of the affected tissues, the prevention of thrombosis and the speeding up of the development of collateral circulation. Remember, there are more than thirty-five papers confirming the effectiveness of alpha tocopherol in the treatment of intermittent claudication.

Alpha tocopherol may also slow up the arteriosclerotic process in the affected vessels or even slightly reverse it, as noted by Boyd and as some retinal studies have suggested. However, as I pointed out in the last chapter, there is now greatly increased hope for the sufferer from arteriosclerosis, whatever its site, in the combination of Vitamin E and Vitamin C. The work which demonstrated this beyond cavil, as you will remember, used 1,200 IU of alpha tocopherol and 3 to 5 gm of ascorbic acid daily. Intravenous chelation with EDTA is also helpful and Vitamins A and D should probably be added.

REFERENCES

1. Begg, T.B. and Richards, R.L. *Scottish Medical Journal* 7/8, 341, 1951.
2. Kannel, W.B., Skinner, J.J., Schwartz, M.J. and Shurtleff, D. *Circulation* 61, 875, 1970.
3. Hacker, R.W. and Decker, R. *Deutsche Medizinische Wochenschrift* 93, 1343, 1968.
4. Myers, K.A. and Irvine, W.J. *British Medical Journal* 1, 879, 1966.
5. Otteman, M.G. and Stahlgren, L.H. *Surgery, Gynecology and Obstetrics* 120, 1217, 1965.
6. Boyd, A.M., Ratcliffe, A.H., Jepson, R.P. and James, G.W.H. *British Journal of Bone and Joint Surgery* 31, 325, 1949.
7. Boyd, A.M., Ratcliffe, A.H., Jepson, R.P. and James, G.W.H. *The Lancet* 2, 132, 1949.
8. Livingstone, P.D. and Jones, C. *The Lancet* 2, 602, 1958.
9. Boyd, A.M. *Angiology* 14, 198, 1963.
10. Larsen, O.A. and Lassen, N.A. *The Lancet* 2, 1093, 1966.

12

THROMBOPHLEBITIS AND PULMONARY EMBOLISM

IN ADDITION TO THE EPIDEMIC of clots in the coronary arteries, there is now an epidemic of clotting in other major and minor vessels.

To state it simply, as I have in Chapter 3, the blood inside all blood vessels must remain fluid at all times, except where there is localized rupture or severing of vessels. Then a thrombus must eventually plug the severed end to stop the loss of blood or, if the vessel is surgically tied off, a clot must form just proximal to the suture. In either case, the clot will be organized and replaced by scar tissue eventually.

However, surgical procedures and many medical conditions, particularly those accompanied by prolonged bed rest, expose many patients to intravenous thrombosis with or without accompanying inflammation. Some operative procedures seem to be particularly likely to produce deep vein thrombosis. Also, the pre-existence of varicose veins with slowing of the return flow of blood or in some areas actual retrograde flow, predisposes the patient to superficial intravenous clots.

Usually, the term *phlebothrombosis* is used to denote the simple intravenous thrombus; the term *thrombophlebitis* suggests a clot in the vein surrounded by an inflammatory reaction.

Using a sensitive test involving radioactive fibrinogen (a coagulant) to detect early thrombosis in the deep veins of the legs, Dr. V. Kakkar of London, England has demonstrated the condition in approximately 28 percent of surgical, 54 percent of orthopedic and 24 percent of urological patients and in 38 percent of patients with myocardial infarction.

Apart from the disturbance of tissues in the area of the involved vein, there is, of course, a definite risk that the thrombus or part of it will break loose, ascend to the right side of the heart and be passed into the pulmonary arteries. When it does, half the patients so afflicted die.

That pulmonary embolism is increasing has been documented. It was reported (1) in 1963 that in two Oxford, England hospitals the incidence of pulmonary embolism increased five times in the period 1952 to 1961. In this series medical cases were more vulnerable than surgical ones. And the use of oral contraceptives increased the incidence of thromboembolic disease from an average of five cases per hundred thousand population in 1967 to forty-seven per hundred thousand in 1968, according to a report in the *British Medical Journal* by Drs. M.P. Vessey and R. Doll in 1969.

Massive acute pulmonary embolism is very difficult to diagnose, the signs and symptoms being deceivingly nonspecific. Therefore, prophylaxis (prevention of the thrombophlebitis) is of the greatest importance.

Many methods have been employed in attempts to prevent the formation of thrombosis at surgery. Because previous studies had shown a risk of 39 percent in hip surgery, Dr. E.W. Saltzman and associates at Harvard Medical School (2) tested the relative effectiveness of four different regimens to prevent thromboembolism. Although their series was small, they were able to report in 1971 that by using aspirin and dextran they had reduced the incidence somewhat—from 39 percent to 12 to 14 percent—still a distressingly high proportion. Another drug, Persantin (dipyridamole), was not very effective and had to be discontinued because of neutropenia (a decrease in the neutrophile white blood cells), dermatitis or severe headache in some subjects.

Moreover, according to the Saltzman group, 3 to 4 percent of the patients treated with anticoagulants, aspirin or dextran had major bleeding complications and patients in the aspirin-treated group required almost twice as much transfused blood as those in the other three groups.

It was reported in 1972 by Dr. J. Bonnar and J. Walsh (3), two English surgeons, that British Dextran 70, administered during and immediately after operation for six hours (started with the anesthetic) produced a "highly significant" reduction in the frequency of thrombosis after abdominal and vaginal hysterectomy for benign conditions.

Another English group used pneumatic leggings to prevent thrombosis in surgical patients. The pneumatic leggings are placed over the feet and lower legs at the time of preoperative anesthesia and are left on until the patient is ambulatory. An electric pump inflates the leggings for one minute followed by one minute of relaxation. The incidence of deep vein thrombosis was 39 percent in those without malignancy who were not using the leggings as against 3 percent in those with the leggings. In cases of malignancy the leggings were of no benefit; about one-half of these patients developed thrombosis.

A 1968 report by Dr. A.M. Antlitz and associates (4) in the United States showed that 32 percent of pulmonary embolism occurred in the first four days after surgery and stated that routine anticoagulant therapy was of no benefit in preventing this.

Thromboembolism is also a risk in obstetrical work. Maternal age, particularly over thirty-five years, and the need for assisted delivery, especially cesarean section, are the most significant factors. Here again, the dangers of estrogen are obvious since its use to inhibit lactation after delivery increases the risk. At age twenty-five and older, the incidence of thromboembolism is doubled if delivery is assisted, even if the patient is lactating. If lactation is suppressed, the risk is increased three times, even with a normal delivery, and at least six times, possibly twelve times, if delivery is assisted, according to a paper by Dr. V.R. Tindall (5) published in 1968.

The extent of the aftermath in the survivors of thromboembolism staggers the imagination. In the United States there are six to seven million patients with severe post-thrombotic symptoms. In Sweden, 1.9 to 3.1 percent of the population are affected and 94 percent of these have sequelae (morbid consequences) with fully 20 percent developing leg ulcers. According to Dr. Haeger (6), the economic importance of these symptoms is higher than that of diabetes mellitus, rheumatism and traffic accidents combined.

The most common end results of phlebitis are edema, varicosities and ulcerations. Among 150 patients followed by Dr. G. Strenger (7) from five to more than twenty years after the initial illness, twenty-five had recurrences. (This was reported in the *New York Journal of Medicine* in 1962.)

Apparently all this is virtually unnecessary. Thrombophlebitis and pulmonary embolism are almost completely preventable. We showed that fresh thrombi could be dissolved completely without the danger of pulmonary embolism in 1946 but could not get this published until 1948. In the same year, as I have mentioned, Zierler and his associates showed that alpha tocopherol was vigorously antithrombic both in vivo and in vitro. Indeed, they proved that it was antithrombic when in normal concentration in human blood.

Since then, there have been fifty-seven papers confirming our work, originating in various foreign countries and in the United States. Since using alpha tocopherol Ochsner has stated as recently as 1968 that he has had no cases of pulmonary embolism.

Not only can fresh thrombophlebitis be melted away —and Ochsner reported in 1950 that he had done this—and pulmonary embolism prevented, but the sequelae can also be completely prevented. Moreover, in cases not so treated in time which therefore have gone on to chronicity with resulting decreased circulation and all that that implies, alpha tocopherol can very greatly diminish the signs and symptoms. Its use in such cases has also been widely confirmed—by Castagna and Impallomeni (8), Mantero et al. (9) and Sturup (10). Confirmation of this has also come from Drs. W.E. Crump and E.F. Heiskell (11), who also confirmed the Ochsner group's results, as did Dr. Terrell Speed.

Suffice it to say, by way of summary, that

1. Thrombosis, arterial or venous, is the Number One Killer in the medical world.
2. Arterial thrombosis, cerebral, coronary and peripheral, is increasing rapidly.
3. Thrombophlebitis and pulmonary embolism are increasing rapidly.
4. A complete answer to some of these problems and a worthwhile answer to most of the others has been known since 1946.

My own experience often illustrates how simple it all could be. On one occasion, a woman came up to me at a dog show and said she had seen me on television. She apparently had seen me on the Merv Griffin Show which had been taped in 1973 in which I, with others, had been discussing preventive medicine, the others being four very distinguished men, Drs. Carlton Fredericks, Linus Pauling, Roger Williams and William Yudkin. (The response of the public to this broadcast has apparently been enormous. It was presented on more than 560 television stations in the United States and Canada and has been repeated at least twice since its original exposure in October, 1973.)

The lady who mentioned this event to me said that she had had to stop indulging in her lifetime hobby of exhibiting show dogs because of disabling phlebitis. After hearing my presentation on television she had gone out to the kennel and taken away the dogs' Vitamin E and taken it herself. She said she needed it more than they did! (Vitamin E is seen as essential to the health of show dogs in many kennels.) The result was great improvement in her legs and a return to active participation in the show ring.

This is but one of hundreds of such cases. The inference is obvious. This woman treated her serious, disabling condition herself so much better than her physician had been able to do. She used Vitamin E. He should have done so—he had no excuse for not doing so—but didn't.

My younger daughter, who is a public health nurse, has quietly suggested Vitamin E treatment to friends when the occasion arose. Here are excerpts from a letter which tells of one such instance and which was in a nutrition magazine, without my daughter's knowledge.

> I am 68 years young, have been troubled with a blood clot in my right leg and it was quite unbearable

at times as I am very active and on my feet almost all day long.

Through very good fortune I happened to rent a suite to a Miss Karen Shute—her father being the author of *Vitamin E for Ailing and Healthy Hearts*, Dr. W.E. Shute, M.D. I started Vitamin E at 800 IU per day since January 1st and in less than eight days the ache and fatigue had left me completely. I really was amazed at the results.

However, before Easter, I ran out of my Vitamin E and two or three days later the old trouble returned, which was at least a good test, so am now convinced that I must take them regularly. I started again and am completely relieved once more.

Had it not been for Miss K. Shute, I would still be ignorant of this "miracle Vitamin E" and still suffering with my ailment.

Mrs. Yvette R. Chapman,
Powell River, B.C.
Canada

A letter received in February 1973 reports as follows:

Your book *Vitamin E for Ailing and Healthy Hearts* has been read with great interest and personally have a phlebitis condition in both legs for a period of over 12 years I was ready to give Vitamin E its trial as after several hospitalizations and all the regular treatments, my legs were getting progressively worse.

I have been on a dosage of 1800 units for a period of 3 months now and remarkedly there is less pain, little or none of the hot spots, and very slight edema compared to much edema by noon everyday.

All this while I have been under the care of . . . an

internist who is beginning to show great interest in my progress. He has asked me to get any literature available on Vitamin E.

REFERENCES

1. *Canadian Medical Association Journal* 89, 1300, 1963.
2. Salzman, E.W., Harris, W.H. and DeSanctis, R.W. *New England Journal of Medicine,* 284, 128, 1971.
3. Bonnar, J. and Walsh, J. *The Lancet* 1, 614, 1972.
4. Antlitz, A.M., Valle, N.G. and Kosai, M.F. *Southern Medical Journal* 61, 307, 1968.
5. Tindall, T.R. *Journal of Obstetrics and Gynaecology of the British Commonwealth* 75, 1324, 1968.
6. Haeger, Knüt. *Angiology* 18, 439, 1968.
7. Strenger, G. *New York Journal of Medicine* 62, 3424, 1962.
8. *Bolletino della Societa Piemont Chirurgia* 18, 155, 1948.
9. *Atti del Congresso di Cardiologia* (Stresa) May, 1949.
10. *Nordisk Medicin* 43, 721, 1950.
11. Crump, W.E. and Heiskell, E.F. *Texas State Journal of Medicine* 41, 11, 1952.

13

HYPERTENSION, STROKES
AND CEREBRAL HEMORRHAGE

SOME TIME AGO, *Time* magazine, in reporting a New York Heart Association conference, presented an excellent summary of the status of hypertension. *Time* quoted Dr. George A. Perera of Columbia University, who had sifted the evidence and studied nearly three thousand patients with primary hypertension, as stating that he had reached a set of conclusions which included the following:

> Victims have many common characteristics, and eventually develop organic complications that cut their life expectancy by as much as 20 years.
> Heredity is vital. "If either mother or father has it, you can bet your boots that at least one of any large family they produce will eventually become hypertensive; and if both parents have it, the majority of their offspring will be afflicted."

Personality stress and diet do not cause the disease, though they may act as triggers for it. Pregnancy and the menopause have little to do with it.

In 1956, for the first time, it became possible to control the blood pressure in the majority of hypertensive patients with little discomfort or inconvenience. What was introduced in that year was the thiazide group of drugs. Hollander and Williams, and Dr. E.D. Freis and his group, soon found that chlorothiazide was as effective or more so in hypertension than diets severely restricted in salt, as well as being more acceptable to the patient. In addition, the chlorothiazide group of drugs greatly enhanced the action of other antihypertensive agents.

Subsequently Freis was able to demonstrate that even moderate hypertension is dangerous and should and can be treated successfully. The results of a five-year, seventeen-hospital study established two main points:

1. Drug treatment for moderate hypertension reduced the death rate by more than 50 percent.
2. Drug treatment is 67 percent effective in preventing major complications which included, among others, strokes, congestive heart failure and kidney failure.

Of course, these same conditions arise in normotensive people as well, but the increased danger in the patient with hypertension is very real.

This is stressed here because one of the beneficial effects of alpha tocopherol on the human heart is its ability to improve the force of contraction of heart muscle, and this may increase the hypertension in roughly one-third of hypertensive patients with cardiac involvement. Small dosage ranges of alpha tocopherol tend to drop the blood pressure in hypertensive patients by decreasing the spasm of end vessels and so decreasing the peripheral resistance.

In the early days of alpha tocopherol therapy of cardiac conditions, the hypertensive patient was often untreatable, since the dangers of a further elevation of his blood pressure outweighed the physicians' desire to treat him with alpha tocopherol. Thus, an adequate dose of alpha tocopherol could not be given to correct angina, congestive failure, peripheral edema and certain other conditions in many patients.

All this changed with the introduction of the chlorothiazides and other antihypertensive drugs. It is now possible in most cases by the judicious use of these drugs plus a carefully selected initial level of alpha tocopherol, raised as the hypertension comes under control, to reach an adequate and effective level of treatment. Caution is still advised.

In spite of constant warnings concerning the danger of large doses of alpha tocopherol in the hypertensive, this remains an area in which full realization of the problem seems very hard to impress on physicians. It is therefore noteworthy that the "authorities" on the use of antihypertensive drugs are having the same difficulties, even eighteen years after effective treatment was established. A survey (1) reported in the *Journal of the American Medical Association* in 1971 showed lack of interest in and neglect of the use of these drugs by physicians, and this was emphasized by an editorial (2) that appeared in the same issue. Says the editorial: "Although these facts seemingly have been well publicized to medical and nonmedical audiences, messages must have been jammed . . . [and] hypertensive patients who would have benefited from therapy were not receiving it."

It must be emphasized as strongly as possible here that the hypertensive patient placed on alpha tocopherol therapy must have simultaneous treatment of his hypertension. Fortunately, just as the chlorothiazides are synergistic with (enhance the action of) other drugs, so alpha tocopherol usually enhances their effect, with excellent control of the blood pressure and the cardiac condition.

Hypertension affects almost twenty-three million Americans. And hypertension is said to be the leading cause of strokes, which kill more than two hundred thousand Americans a year and thus are the third leading cause of death.

Interestingly enough, although deaths from coronary artery disease or myocardial infarction have increased rapidly in the last sixty years, there is every reason to believe that there has been no significant alteration in the incidence of cerebral hemorrhage or thrombosis during this period. This, of course, confirms the observations of Dr. J.N. Morris of England, Dr. Hans Nieper of Germany and others that there has been little change in the prevalence of atherosclerosis during the same sixty-year period. This is confirmed in a paper in *The Lancet* by Drs. T.W. Anderson and J.S. MacKay (3).

I should like to make three observations in passing.

First, for those physicians who insist on double-blind controlled experiments, the article by Fries in the *Journal of the American Medical Association* in 1971 that I have already mentioned suggests they may never be justified. In a controlled trial of various suggested antihypertensive drugs the trial was terminated "after only 18 months of treatment because of the great difference in morbidity and mortality in the control vs. the treated patients." Had this been a "double-blind" it would not have been discovered until the project had been completed that the deaths were occurring chiefly in the control group.

Second, I should like to point out that the absence of an increase in the incidence of cerebral accidents, in contrast with the rapid and steady increase in coronary thrombosis and myocardial infarction, is further evidence that the oft-repeated concept that thrombosis occurs because of atherosclerotic changes in the vessel wall is just not so.

Finally, I should like to remind my readers of a factor in

the hypertension picture that relates back to the estrogens, the work on which was actually the basis for all of our work on the use of alpha tocopherol. As we have already seen, estrogens and alpha tocopherol are antagonistic. This concept, long resisted by the profession, has now been largely confirmed by the increasing evidence that the oral contraceptives are responsible for an increase in hypertension and in intravascular clotting. The resulting hypertension is usually curable by stopping "the pill."

As for treatment of stroke victims, apparently there isn't any—except for alpha tocopherol. According to the *Medical Post* (8 December 1970), Dr. H.J.M. Barnett, speaking at the annual meeting of the Ontario Chapter of the College of Family Physicians of Canada, had this to say: "As of this minute there is nothing, nothing, absolutely nothing that will improve cerebral blood circulation. I was at a meeting last month where all the experts from the world on cerebral circulation were gathered—75 of them—and the unanimous conclusion was that everything [in this field] that was being pushed by the drug companies was absolutely worthless."

The patients we have seen over the past twenty-seven years have come, as I have said before, from many different and widely scattered places in the world as well as from those cities in which we practice. There has, therefore, been a predominance of chronic cases over acute, although we have had a great many of both. There has not been, proportionately, a large number of cerebral accident cases. They probably, on the whole, constitute the single group in which treatment with alpha tocopherol is least satisfactory.

In contrast with the person who has survived a myocardial infarction, who usually can be maintained for years in apparently normal health or nearly so, the help alpha tocopherol can give to the stroke patient is much more limited. The reason is obvious, of course. Since the various areas of the brain have their specific functions and pathways, once an area dies and liquifies, its functions are lost forever. In comparison the post-infarct patient is fortunate. As long as the walls of the chambers of the heart are intact and provided that the blood supply to the heart muscle that is left is adequate, the organ works as a whole unit. Even a large area of infarction, once healed, may not adversely affect the action of the whole organ.

Nevertheless, alpha tocopherol will help most stroke victims because of its two principal functions: reducing the oxygen need of living tissue and preventing fresh thrombi. Whether alpha tocopherol has the ability to remove a fresh thrombus in a cerebral artery if given at the onset of symptoms is certainly debatable, but it is quite possible that it does have this power. However, the brain cells are so sensitive to anoxia that it is certainly still a critical situation. In general, alpha tocopherol will help to this degree if the patient survives: the patient who is bedfast will improve to the point at which he can be promoted to a chair; the chair patient will usually be able to walk with help whether it be a cane or crutch; and the patient on cane or crutch can usually walk unaided. However, complete recovery is never possible, and it is pathetic to see a man who has been helped to a certain degree hope and struggle to achieve still further help from alpha tocopherol.

The chance of recurrence, however, is greatly reduced by alpha tocopherol, although in severe cases this is not necessarily desirable from the point of view of the patient or his family. Some of these patients are pathetic in their need for constant care and supervision; some are so grossly unhappy, some are mere vegetables.

Around the area of heart muscle that is deprived of blood supply in a heart attack, as around the area of softening in the brain after a stroke, is a zone of varying width in which the cells have almost, but not quite, died. This is commonly called the "zone of injury." At the time of the attack or stroke it barely received enough blood from a neighboring artery to allow its cells to survive. Around this zone is another, also of varying width, which did get some blood from the blocked vessel but more of its supply from the adjacent vessels. This is usually called the "zone of anoxia." It is these two zones which are helped by alpha tocopherol. If they are of considerable extent, then the patient will show definite and worthwhile clinical improvement. If they are relatively narrow, the improvement will be less obvious.

Alpha tocopherol is effective in treating stroke patients in the way that I have just described where the lesion is an embolus or cerebral artery thrombosis. It is not effective in cases of cerebral hemorrhage, of course. This is one group of patients that no one likes to treat since the brain is so sensitive to depletion of oxygen, and brain tissue, once dead, is irreplaceable.

As in the myocardial infarct and the stroke caused by thrombosis, there are two zones surrounding the necrotic (dead) area of softening produced by a cerebral accident that are not functioning normally. One is called, once again, the area of injury, the other the area of anoxia. Again, alpha tocopherol improves the performance of the nerve cells in these two areas. When these areas are large and where they involve cells with important specific functions, the result of treatment can be worthwhile. The ideal situation consists of a small area of necrosis with a large zone of living but not functioning cells surrounding it. The most unsatisfactory group of patients are those with large areas of softening with minimal zones of injury and anoxia.

The result that can usually be expected is, once again, the promotion of the patient to the next stage of improvement. If he is a bed patient, he will very likely be able to be cared for in a chair as well. His control of excretory functions will improve and he may be much easier to look after. The chair patient can usually learn to get around with help and crutches. The crutch patient can usually graduate to a cane, and the man who uses a cane can usually discard it.

However, I have had so many of these "cerebral accident" patients under my care that I am used to the usual reaction: hope and happiness at first and an expectation of continuous improvement, which indeed occurs for some months but which so often falls short of the hoped-for end result.

Almost surely, vigorous and continuous physiotherapy, and especially brain-retraining techniques, could extend the degree of improvement, but this is difficult to obtain for the patient since hospitals and physiotherapists have long been conditioned to viewing these patients with pessimism, expecting them to suffer a recurrence and therefore not to be worth persistent efforts at rehabilitation.

The protective action of Vitamin E in preventing a subsequent attack, then, is a double-edged sword. It prolongs the months or years during which the seriously handicapped patients must be cared for without offering additional help. This, of course, does not apply to the victim who recovers nearly completely from the cerebral accident, who is able to take care of himself normally and who has no diminution of his mental capacities. This patient should have 1,600 IU of alpha tocopherol a day, excepting always the patients with the two complications in which it is not safe to use so large a dose—hypertension and chronic rheumatic heart disease.

REFERENCES

1. *Journal of the American Medical Association* 218, 1036, 1971.
2. *Journal of the American Medical Association* 218, 1043, 1971.
3. Anderson, T.W. and MacKay, J.S. *The Lancet* 1, 1136, 1968.

14

DIABETES MELLITUS

MY YOUNGER DAUGHTER has a co-worker in the public health unit of a western Canadian city who has a severe case of diabetes. All women diabetics go on to severe premature arteriosclerotic changes. This nurse had reached the stage at which she had gross symptoms of these changes in her eyes and her legs and feet. One toe had shown discoloration, and the blood supply of both legs and feet was seriously reduced. They were cold and numb and she had reached the so-called pregangrenous state. After my daughter told her some of the facts about alpha tocopherol, she started to take it and her condition has improved to an amazing degree.

Remember that this woman is a very intelligent nurse, that she understands diabetes mellitus and that she has been constantly checked by physicians for many years. The simple addition of alpha tocopherol is, therefore, the sole reason for her improvement. Incidentally, she is one of the 30 percent of diabetics whose insulin requirements drop. She now takes about half of her former dose and she is much better controlled and stabilized than she was.

Elsewhere I have related the case of a woman doctor, English by birth and training, who practiced in Ireland. She developed diabetes mellitus, then hypertension, then angina and then had a myocardial infarction. She was treated in England for all these conditions but had to retire. A chance consultation about her dog with Dr. N.H. Lambert of Dublin, then president of the Irish Veterinary Association and a man who is very familiar with the actions of Vitamin E in his practice, led her to take an adequate dose of synthetic alpha tocopherol. The result was a disappearance of all angina, a return of her blood pressure to normal, a reduction of her insulin requirement and finally a return to active practice.

When this woman visited me she ended the consultation by asking why she, a physician acquainted with many other physicians, had had to learn the secret of successful treatment of her own case from her veterinarian!

I mention these two cases because they concern a nurse and a highly trained doctor, both of whom are familiar with diabetes and its serious consequences.

Diabetes is another cardiovascular disease which is increasing rapidly worldwide. In some countries, reports the World Health Organization, the death rate is two or three times higher than it was ten years ago.

Once again, the reasons that alpha tocopherol is useful in the treatment of diabetes are its specific actions in assisting the tissues that are affected by the blood vessel changes characteristic of the disease. Alpha tocopherol can decrease the oxygen need of tissues, it can prevent thrombosis and it can accelerate the development of collateral circulation. The decrease in insulin dosage in about one-third of the cases is an incidental benefit.

There are now forty-six papers in the medical literature confirming the value of alpha tocopherol in the treatment of diabetes mellitus.

The vascular complications of diabetes involve brain, eye, heart, kidney and extremities. Insulin, hailed as a wonderful discovery in 1921, has saved many lives and has prolonged by many years comparatively normal health in the victims of this disease. It was not at first realized, however, that diabetes was not only an abnormality of carbohydrate metabolism but a disease affecting the whole cardiovascular system. The result, therefore, of the control of the former by insulin was the prolongation of life to the stage at which the seriousness of the cardiovascular changes became evident. These changes are usually generalized, and when the blood supply becomes decreased in the legs to a point at which symptoms begin, there is usually associated coronary or cerebral artery disease.

Diabetic gangrene leads to amputation, first of one leg and then the other. In one orthopedic service at the University of Miami School of Medicine, Dr. Augusto Sarmiento reported that of more than two hundred diabetic patients requiring amputation of an ischemic (blood-starved) leg about 50 percent required amputation of the remaining leg within two years.

This is a sad commentary on diabetic treatment with insulin and diet. In our practice we regularly salvage such legs even with the toes completely necrotic. We have saved legs in which the gangrene was infected and extended into the metatarsal area of the foot and in one case where the whole heel pad was involved. We have colored slides to prove the success of this treatment in such extreme cases.

All diabetics must have a measure of dietary control, and insulin if this is also necessary, that will keep the blood sugar within reasonable bounds. They also must have alpha tocopherol to prevent the serious effects of arteriosclerosis. And it begins to appear that of equal importance is 3 to 5 gm of ascorbic acid daily.

Until alpha tocopherol is added to the treatment of every diabetic patient, unnecessary loss of life, amputations, blindness, hypertension and myocardial infarction will continue to be the lot of more and more diabetics.

15

VITAMIN E OINTMENT IN BURNS AND OTHER CONDITIONS

THAT EVERY CELL IN THE BODY must have Vitamin E is now firmly established. That the body needs many essential nutrients, amino acids, minerals and thirteen vitamins is now accepted by every biochemist. (The authority on this is Roger Williams, B.S., M.S., Ph.D., D.Sc. I recommend his book *Nutrition Against Disease* as a nutritional bible.)

That oxygen directly applied to damaged tissues can initiate and promote healing has also been well established. Hyperbaric oxygen applied locally can effectively shorten healing time in most chronic leg ulcers as well as in many decubitus ulcers. (Anyone who is interested in this form of treatment should consult the article by Dr. B.H. Fisher (1) in *The Lancet.*)

Alpha tocopherol acts in a different manner to accomplish the same purpose, but has the advantage of acting not only locally as the pure oil or in an ointment base, but also systematically through the blood supply to the cell. It is not surprising, therefore, that by far the best treatment for burns is alpha tocopherol orally and by direct application.

The efficacy of alpha tocopherol is well illustrated by the experience of one of my nurses. This twenty-four-year-old very blonde nurse lay out in the sun on the beach on the first beautiful spring day. She was clad in a relatively scant bathing suit. She fell asleep and overstayed a reasonable time of exposure to the sun. The result was an intense sunburn over her face and neck and all the areas not covered by the bathing suit. She attempted to work the next morning but was nauseated and weak. She was brought to me by her co-worker in the electrocardiograph and laboratory division of the Shute Institute. She was running a fever, had a severe headache and was a very sick-looking girl.

Conventional treatment would probably have prescribed for her compresses of boric acid, doses of antihistamine, cor-ticosteroid spray or cream and possibly painkiller medication.

We put this nurse in one of the side rooms, covered all the burned areas liberally with Vitamin E ointment and covered her with a sheet. Within minutes she fell asleep. Within an hour her temperature was normal and her headache had vanished. She got up and went back to work.

Our nurse did not develop a single blister and she did not peel. This is all the more remarkable since it was about twenty hours after the burn that treatment was initiated.

Earlier I have related the unblind controlled experiment of a man familiar with the value of Vitamin E and Vitamin E ointment in treating burns. He applied the ointment to half the burn, and the difference between the two areas was obvi-ous and striking. The owner of a company which wholesales Vitamin E products used the same technique on a severe

barbecue burn on his thumb. The difference between the
E-ointment-treated part of the burn and the other half was
very obvious.

As I write this, my wife has suggested that I mention her
ninety-one-year-old mother who, apart from some loss of
hearing, is able to do all that the average sixty-year-old can
do. She swims miles every day in the summer and is in the
pool at least once a day when we are in Florida. She should be
long since dead, for she had hypertension for years, developed a bundle branch block and then the dyspnea of congestive failure. Control of her hypertension with diuretics and
2,400 IU of alpha tocopherol a day, however, keep her well
and vigorous.

Some six or seven years ago my mother-in-law acciden-
tally upset a dish of boiling water on her foot which was in a
sock and slipper. The whole dorsum was involved in a deep
burn. Vitamin E ointment was applied within seconds, and
today there is no visible trace of the burn.

Vitamin E has no equal for first- and second-degree
burns and is a useful adjunctive therapy in third-degree
burns. It has three unique characteristics. First, it lessens or
takes away the associated pain a few minutes after application. Second, it keeps the burn from deepening, limiting the
damage to the cells actually destroyed by the burning agent.
Finally, it gives rapid epithelization and a scar that is not
painful and does not contract. (Because it is antibacterial in
vivo and in vitro, incidentally, it virtually removes the danger
of infection.)

The majority of burn patients treated in this way do not
need hospitalization. More important is the great reduction in
the need for skin grafting. It is seldom necessary even in
severe third-degree burns. Because the scars do not contract,
there are no contraction deformities when the burns involve

the axilla (armpit) or neck or groin. The color slides we show at medical conferences of the results of treating burns are unique and completely convincing.

The late Adelle Davis (2), reported remarkable case histories emphasizing the value of tocopherol in the healing of burns without scars. Vitamin E, in fact, is such a useful product for domestic burns and sunburns that many who are familiar with it keep a tube in several rooms in the house, especially the kitchen, and never travel without it.

Vitamin E ointment has many uses in addition to its major role in the treatment of burns.* It was first used in the treatment of ulcerations on the legs due to venous stasis (stagnation) or arterial insufficiency. These ulcers healed well with oral Vitamin E, but in most cases more rapidly with the addition of the local application of the ointment. However, the scars formed in these ulcer cases were surprising. They were the same size as the original ulcers, and they were soft, pliable and not tender.

When Vitamin E ointment is used on scars following abdominal surgery they will often virtually disappear. The ointment is especially useful after radical mastectomy, particularly where there is superficial irritation due to radiation. It not only reduces the toxic reactions but soothes and heals the irritated areas.

Vitamin E ointment is also useful on acne scars and on scars about the face due to lacerations from windshield glass in automobile accidents. Not long ago my two-year-old grandson, standing up on the front seat of the car, was precipitated onto the rear view mirror. An elliptical piece of skin approximately 1 by 2 cm from his forehead was left on the mirror.

* For an account of the effectiveness of oral and local alpha tocopherol in more severe cases, see the chapter on burns in *Vitamin E for Ailing and Healthy Hearts*.

My grandson was seen very soon afterward by his local general practitioner. The doctor told my daughter to bring him the piece of skin. He washed it in saline and sewed it into the defect—an amazingly dextrous job on a two-year-old since he had, of course, to tease the contracted piece of skin back into approximately normal size and shape.

I chanced to arrive on the scene on the day the stitches were removed, and there was certainly grave doubt then that the patch would survive. It was raised in the center and quite inflamed around about half its periphery. As soon as the stitch holes sealed over, Vitamin E ointment was liberally applied with the result that although there was a very small area of superficial necrosis in the center, the cosmetic results six months later were excellent. The patch continues to improve and is now scarcely noticeable. The child's physician does not know the ointment is being used, and my daughter happily relates this excellent physician's surprise at the steady and unexpected improvement.

Vitamin E ointment has another specific use—namely, in the treatment of nerve root pain. Intercostal neuritis or neuralgia, sciatica and various cases of myositis (muscle inflammation) respond to Vitamin E inunction. Drs. Burgess and Pritchard of the Montreal General Hospital long ago reported that Vitamin E could be recovered at the periosteum of bones and joints shortly after the ointment was rubbed into the overlying skin. The ointment, rubbed in gently for ten minutes and followed by the application of heat for ten minutes over the nerve roots of the sensory nerves involved in a neuritis, will relieve the condition in a majority of cases. If it does not do so within one to three nights of application, however, it is unlikely to help.

A great many doctors, especially in Canada, have long scoffed at manipulation. They have given excellent reasons why manipulation cannot help and I expect that this has been taught in every medical school, as it was in mine. However, there is now an association of trained physicians manipulating patients with the various neuritic lesions. Many surgeons attempt manipulation under anesthesia as do many in the new specialty of physical medicine.

About 50 percent of patients who have had myocardial infarcts or angina often also have pains in the chest unrelated to coronary artery disease. The cervical root syndrome closely mimics heart pain. Many of these cases respond to manipulation. Dr. Paul Goodley described such a case at the fifth International Congress of Physical Medicine in 1968. His patient, a fifty-two-year-old longshoreman, had suffered serious neck injuries in a car accident. His severe pain of fifteen months duration was completely relieved by manipulation under anesthesia. Incidentally, this doctor of medicine was refused permission to do this manipulation in his hospital.

At the same meeting Dr. Janet Travell, Associate Clinical Professor of Medicine at George Washington University, and Dr. John Mennell, Associate Professor of Medicine and Rehabilitation at the University of Pennsylvania, reported on the virtues of manipulation. Manipulation can give instant relief from pain and from restriction of movement in some cases.

Vitamin E ointment somehow does the same in most cases of sciatica, intercostal neuralgia, frozen shoulder and others of that type. Many cases of months or years duration respond. When they do not, we have for years sent patients for manipulation with excellent results, again in most cases.

An interesting instance of Vitamin E—but not, apparently, E ointment—helping in a muscular condition, occurred in Chicago. Some years ago, a Chicago newspaper contained an account of an unusual case involving a ten-year-old boy whose leg muscles had become so hard, owing to calcium deposits, that they were described as "turning to stone." The newspaper said that the boy's doctors believed that "highly concentrated doses of Vitamin E" had helped him so that he could walk a few steps. They were, they said, expecting considerably more improvement.

In 1965 Drs. R.H. Brodkin and J. Bleiberg (3) reported that there can be allergic reactions to Vitamin E applied locally. We have noted this from the very beginning of its use and have warned all patients, for years, that about 10 percent of people cannot tolerate the full-strength ointment on open wounds or ulcers. Before it is applied to the whole area, Vitamin E should always be used on one corner of the ulcer or sore until it is evident that it does not cause a local reaction. We first published this caution in 1950.

The ointment is a 30 IU per gm of alpha tocopherol in a petroleum jelly base, and those who cannot tolerate a full-strength ointment can often derive benefit without reaction from a half-strength dilution. If there is still reaction to the local application of the ointment, opening a capsule of the succinate preparation and scattering the powder over the ulcer can often be tolerated and can be very effective.

We decry the use of Vitamin E for any nonmedical reason. We were horrified at its use as a deodorant. Had the companies concerned bothered to consult us, we could have told them that many users would show allergic reactions. However, our main objection arises from the fact that this substance is often in short supply as the result of its rapid acceptance for prophylactic and therapeutic use in medicine. It is a shame to see it wasted.

The mechanism by which the Vitamin E ointment functions is quite unknown and very puzzling. New uses for it, however, keep cropping up constantly. Often we hear about them only by letter. In this connection, let me quote three paragraphs from a letter from a woman in a large mid-western city:

> I was born with a hemangioma (birthmark) on my
> face. It covers my left eye, forehead, cheek, nose

and upper part of my left lip.

As my sister, who is a medical doctor, read your book on Vitamin E, she thought it would be advisable that I take Vitamin E. I started with 400 units for a period of 6 months, then increased to 600, and since August 1973, to date I am taking 800 units per day. The reason my sister recommended that I take Vitamin E was because I had rheumatism when I was 15 years old.

During the first six months I was taking Vitamin E I did not notice any change on my hemangioma but suddenly I started noting that it was fading out little by little and right now it has faded out almost one centimeter all around the birthmark. At the same time that I was taking Vitamin E, my sister ordered from Canada Vitamin E ointment and I applied it on my face with a lamp (200 watts). I think the birthmark started disappearing since I started applying the ointment and taking the Vitamin E. I have applied 3 jars of ointment.

REFERENCES

1. Fisher, B.H. *The Lancet* 2, 405, 1969.
2. Davis, A. *Here's Health* 11, 4, 1967.
3. Brodkin, R.H. and Bleiber, J. *Archives of Dermatology* 92, 76, 1965.

16

TAILORING THE DOSE

IF YOU ARE A DOCTOR and are interested in alpha tocopherol therapy for your patients, you will find in this chapter the information you will need in determining dosage levels for a variety of different kinds of cases. I would suggest that before reading it you should look back at Chapter 7 to review for yourself the material there describing the basic functions of alpha tocopherol and its role in the human body.

Treatment with alpha tocopherol must be tailored to each patient's needs. As with most other potent and useful medications, such as insulin, for example, the dosage level in different individuals with apparently the same signs and symptoms may vary widely. Our motto in this is, "Tailor the dose." And we are constantly mindful of the concept of "biochemical individuality" which I have mentioned previously in connection with Roger Williams. Obviously, too, there are certain precautions to be observed—again, as with any potent medication.

Because alpha tocopherol increases the efficiency of all tissues with its oxygen-sparing ability, it may increase the tone of heart muscle. This is important in hypertension and hypertensive heart disease. In about one-third of hypertensives, it may raise the level of already elevated blood pressure if appropriate antihypertensive drugs are not prescribed at appropriate dosage levels. Fortunately, alpha tocopherol seems to enhance the action of most antihypertensive drugs, and most patients with hypertension respond to treatment for this condition and, having done so, can then be given the same quantity of alpha tocopherol as though they were normotensive.

Inorganic iron destroys the activity of alpha tocopherol when they meet outside or inside the body. If iron must be given, ingestion of the two substances must be separated by eight to twelve hours.

Estrogens and alpha tocopherol are antagonists. Moreover, in most conditions which require alpha tocopherol treatment, the use of estrogens is ineffective or actually contraindicated.

The effect of digitalis on the heart is enhanced by alpha tocopherol. In many patients, the optimum effect of digitalis may be demonstrated at a level between one-half and one-fifth of the dosage used in the same patient before alpha tocopherol was used. Conversely, *if the usual dosage of digitalis is not reduced when the patient is given the optimum dosage of alpha tocopherol, the patient may well be overdigitalized and experience all the symptoms of digitalis poisoning.*

Digitalis should only be used in patients with auricular fibrillation to slow the heart rate to an optimum level. It is obviously impossible to gauge the effect of digitalis on the patient with normal sinus rhythm except when the symptoms of overdosage appear.

According to a report to the Japanese Rheumatism Society by Dr. Takefumi Morotomi and Dr. Sadao Kira, Vitamin E may have striking value for many rheumatoid arthritic patients who require treatment with steroids. Steroids have undesirable side-effects and the addition of Vitamin E allows a reduction of the steroid dosage to one-third with great reduction in side-effects. The doctors cite as a typical case that of a twenty-nine-year-old housewife with arthritis of elbows, arms, fingers and legs who improved on very high steroid doses but deteriorated and became scarcely able to walk on 15 mg of Prednisolene. With Vitamin E therapy added, just 3 mg of the steroid now permits her to be active to the point of enjoying folk dancing and bicycle riding. In addition to its value in increasing steroid activity, the physicians report, Vitamin E stimulates the circulation in the extremities and patients commonly tell of losing the "cold feeling" in their limbs.

Incidentally, Drs. P.M. DeSanctis and G.A. Furey have reported in the *Journal of Urology* some interesting results in the treatment of Peyronie's disease (a condition characterized by painful swelling of the male sex organ). With steroids alone, 85 percent were helped; with steroids and Vitamin E, 100 percent were helped. No other therapy was really useful.

As indicated throughout this book, the use of polyunsaturated fats always increases the need for alpha tocopherol and serves no useful purpose in any case. If patients do not stop following this tragic fad, they will not get the full effect of alpha tocopherol treatment.

Megavitamin ascorbic acid will enhance and improve the patient's response to alpha tocopherol in retinal arteriosclerosis whatever the etiology and in peripheral vascular and coronary artery disease. *However a large quantity of ascorbic acid must not be given to patients with chronic rheumatic heart disease. In this condition, the alpha tocopherol dosage is most critical, and the dosage schedule given later on in this chapter and in Chapter 10 must be adhered to strictly.*

Whereas results of treatment with alpha tocopherol in acute rheumatic fever, acute nephritis and acute thrombophlebitis will usually occur in a matter of days, improvement in coronary disease is rarely noted in less than ten days but is usually obvious in four to six weeks. If such a patient does not respond within six weeks, the dosage must be raised at six-week intervals until he does respond or until it is obvious that he will not. I have seen patients greatly improve on 4,000 IU who showed no improvement on dosages of 800 to 3,200 IU.

As has been mentioned by Boyd, Haeger and others, patients with intermittent claudication may show response only after three months of more of treatment. As a rule, peripheral vascular cases require large daily amounts of alpha tocopherol—more than is required in the average coronary case.

If a chronic rheumatic heart disease patient who has been on Vitamin E for years discontinues his treatment, he may seem as well as ever for some time. In contrast, coronary patients who stop their treatment with alpha tocopherol may have a recurrence of symptoms, or even an occlusion, after three days. The coronary patient must never decrease the level of dosage at which he received definite help nor ever stop for more than two days. If such a patient suffers an accident or is hospitalized for surgery, emergency or elective, he needs his alpha tocopherol more than ever and, if at all possible, must have it. It may be omitted on the day of the operation if absolutely necessary. Of course, as Ochsner has pointed out, all surgical patients should be given alpha tocopherol before and after surgery to prevent thrombophlebitis and pulmonary embolism. For the treated coronary patient, it is doubly important.

Let me now summarize our treatment of various conditions and at the same time indicate the dosage range for alpha tocopherol in each one.

Acute coronary thrombosis. Emergency use of such antispasmodics as intravenous papverine, amyl nitrate "bombs" to attempt to relieve the spasm and the pain, with nitroglycerine as necessary and at least 1,600 IU of alpha tocopherol as soon as possible. Levine's armchair treatment with bathroom privileges as soon as the patient is free of pain, and ambulation after ten days. No anticoagulants ever and no polyunsaturated fats or inorganic iron.

Patients who have survived without the above treatment should be started on 800 to 1,200 IU a day and their status reviewed at six-week intervals. Patients should be maintained indefinitely on the quantity to which they responded. Nitroglycerine should be freely used and hypertension, if present, vigorously treated.

Peripheral vascular conditions. Patients are started on 1,600 IU a day and the dosage increased at six-week intervals. Careful cleanliness of feet and legs is observed in the arterial cases. Patients with varicose ulcers, burns and other open wounds are given 800 to 1,600 IU a day, with simultaneous use of alpha tocopherol ointment. As I have said, about 10 percent will show a local reaction to the ointment but may tolerate half-strength ointment or the succinate powder from a capsule.

Intermittent claudication. Patients should be forced to engage in regular walking exercises, to the utmost extent possible. This, along with 800 to 3,200 IU of Vitamin E, should yield excellent results in virtually every such patient. It is very worthwhile to add 2 to 5 gm of Vitamin C if the patient can tolerate it.

Acute rheumatic fever. Alpha tocopherol dosage here is 800 to 1,200 IU a day.

Chronic rheumatic heart disease. Here alpha tocopherol dosage is 75 IU a day for four weeks with no obvious help, 100 IU a day for four weeks with no obvious help, then 150 IU level. Occasionally a patient may respond at the 100 IU level. (Most will continue to improve on 150 IU a day, and most will regress if given more. Occasionally, after a long time on 150 IU, it may be possible and desirable to very carefully increase the dosage by small increments to a maximum of 300 IU—but more than 300 IU should *absolutely never* be used.)

Before a physician treats a chronic rheumatic heart disease patient with alpha tocopherol he should read carefully the part of this book that deals with this subject (Chapter 9).

I can summarize my beliefs about dosage in one sentence. The important thing in alpha tocopherol therapy is to give enough of a properly labelled and assayed product to do the job, and be sure to observe the restrictions outlined earlier and above.

Recently two letters have appeared in *The Lancet,* both warning against overuse of Vitamin E and claiming that weakness and fatigue are common side-effects of excessive use of Vitamin E. The content of these letters has been disseminated throughout the United States in the press. I mention this here in order to deny categorically the truth of such statements.

Weakness and fatigue are never caused by megavitamin E. It has not been mentioned by a single patient or noted by us in one single patient in the more than twenty-five years of our experience with Vitamin E.

In fact, by improving circulation and the ability of the tissues to make the fullest use of their oxygen supply, Vitamin E has exactly the opposite effect in humans and animals alike.

The doctor using Vitamin E therapy can with absolute safety ignore these "warnings."

17

THE HEALTHY HEART

THE PUBLISHERS CHOSE THE TITLE for *Vitamin E for Ailing and Healthy Hearts.* As a result, many readers must have expected to find in that book some specific mention of the quantity of E intake necessary for the healthy heart. Some of them wrote me to complain that they could not find this information.

I think that it should be obvious to anyone who has read the whole book that no man, woman or child can assume that he or she has a healthy heart. In today's world, Vitamin E deficiency can begin very early in life. And it can get worse as time goes on—very much worse.

Arrayed against each one of us is our great industrialized civilization. No one wants to go back to the "good old days." All of us appreciate the conveniences of modern living. However, there have developed serious dangers in our mode of life—air, water and soil pollution, to mention but a few obvious ones.

More serious is the chemicalization of our foods. The promotion of soft drinks, sugar-containing foods and convenience packaging has changed our eating habits beyond recognition. The point has finally been reached at which most people buy from the supermarkets, and there is scarcely a single product in the store which hasn't been chemically treated. Most milk, bread, canned foods, candy, ice cream and many other items are loaded with chemicals, many of which interfere with adequate nutrition.

The *Journal of the American Medical Association* in 1970 published a report (1) of the Council on Foods and Nutrition to the American Medical Association Board of Trustees in which the woeful state of malnutrition and hunger in the United States is spelled out in detail. "Malnutrition producing physiological impairment seems to be common," say the authors of the report. It was specifically stated in a Department of Agriculture report printed in the same journal (for 19 July 1971) that everyone should use nutritional food supplements.

It requires a real effort to obtain adequate nutrition today. It means avoidance of most of our "treats" and most of our desserts and careful selection and preparation of our fruits and vegetables. It may even mean the return to some of the ways of old—such as, when possible, our own home-raised vegetables and home canning. Most of all, it means finding someone who can give one a complete nutritional checkup and evaluation and then prescribe additions of the appropriate supplements. And such checkups are completely foreign to the medical training of virtually all presently practicing physicians and a far cry from the teachings offered under the heading of "nutrition" in most high schools and colleges.

Treating a "healthy heart" means recognizing the nearly

complete removal of the essential antithrombin from our natural diets and the urgent need for its restoration in much greater quantities than ever needed before—at least 800 IU of alpha tocopherol a day in most adults (probably less in younger people).

Supplementation must begin at birth, assuming the mother was taking enough to keep the baby's level up to normal. It is probably the best insurance, along with Vitamin C, against crib deaths.

Apparently not all infants have enough alpha tocopherol. An article (2) in the *New England Journal of Medicine* reports a case of coronary thrombosis with resulting death in a premature infant who died 18 hours after birth. "Coronary occlusion with myocardial infarction has been reported in several instances in patients of the 'newborn' and childhood age groups."

Babies should not have less than 30 IU a day, more as they grow older. It is only the newborn who have any chance of maintaining a normal level throughout life.

For the rest of us, it is too late to achieve a "healthy heart." We have been deprived of an absolutely essential food element by the wonders of the modern technologies of the manufacturers of most of our flour, bread, cereals and other convenience foods.

A startling example of this deprivation has come to light through investigative activities of the National Aeronautical and Space Administration (NASA).

A Canadian scientist, Dr. David Turner, who was one of the first developers of gas chromatography (an analytic process in which gases or vapors are separated) and who because of his expertise in the use of this process was associated with the astronaut program, stated in a television interview that the loss by the American spacemen of up to 20 percent of their red blood cells was probably caused by a lack of Vitamin E in their food. As Turner said on television, he had been led to suspect that lack of E was the culprit because of his familiarity with the work of the Shute brothers—a familiarity he had acquired while working in London, Ontario. On Apollo Ten and subsequent flights the astronauts have had their freeze-dried foods fortified with Vitamin E and on these trips they have suffered no red cell loss. On the earlier flights in which red cell loss had occurred, the result was considerable fatigue.

The civilian application is obvious. Freeze-dried convenience foods are coming into general use and they will have to have their Vitamin E restored or hemolytic anemia could become more prevalent.

I received a letter about the astronauts' diet from Houston, Texas in January, 1970. It was actually a copy of the one written to the Editor of *Prevention* and since it was meant for publication and information I shall give you excerpts from it:

My sister and I subscribe to *Prevention* and live by the *Prevention* system. She works at the Manned Spacecraft Center (NASA) near Houston, in the bio-medical division directly for the doctors, planning the diets of the astronauts. Because of her, Vitamin E, calcium and other supplements have been added to the diets of the astronauts. She constantly put your *Prevention* articles under the noses of the doctors until it brought results. You may give yourself credit for this. Dr. Shute was wondering how this came about (*Vitamin E for Ailing and Healthy Hearts*, Dec., 1969) so I'm enclosing a copy of this letter for him.

My sister answers the phone at NASA "Food and Nutrition." She was picked to work in Mission Control during the first landing on the moon. The heartbeat, etc. of the astronauts was constantly monitored, and it is interesting to note that when they stepped on the moon their pulse rate almost doubled.

This is really not a new discovery although Dr. Turner apparently was not aware that the Aerospace Medical Association at a Miami meeting on 13 May 1964 decided that every explorer going out into space should be fortified with a diet high in Vitamin E. This was published in *Aerospace Medicine* for September 1964 but apparently ignored for some time.

It is strange that while starvation has always elicited interest, malnutrition has, in the past at least, attracted almost no attention at all. In 1974, however, a new campaign was launched with considerable fanfare to improve the nutrition of the American consumer, particularly the young girl. Television spots are being used and a book entitled *Food Is More Than Just Something to Eat* is being distributed free to those who write in for it. This is part of a new Advertising Council campaign launched with the help of the United States government and the food industry. The book was prepared with help from the U.S. Department of Agriculture and the U.S. Department of Health, Education and Welfare. The campaign was launched by Virginia Knauer, Special Assistant to the President for Consumer Affairs.

Mrs. Knauer has been quoted as saying that the public needs to have a far greater awareness of nutrition and that poor nutrition is common in the United States. "The percentage of households that meet or exceed the U.S. Department of Agriculture's definition of a good diet dropped from 60 to 50 percent between 1955 and 1965 . . . Even many relatively affluent individuals have poor diets." Mrs. Knauer evinced concern about "the mounting cost of diet-related illnesses [and of] remedial education required to overcome diet-related slowness in school. . . ."

This is at least a beginning. Another good sign is that nutrition is an area in which many doctors are now for the first time beginning to take an interest.

Knowledge of nutrition has been hard to come by, since until very recently the subject was not a part of the medical student's curriculum. As recently as 1970 there was no course in nutrition taught in any of our medical schools. All the doctor-to-be was taught was that there were three classes of foods—protein, carbohydrate and fat—and a few substances called vitamins that in minute quantities were essential for adequate nutrition. His knowledge of vitamins consisted of the information that their absence could cause some rather exotic conditions such as scurvy (a full-blown case of which he would never see), beriberi (which only a Southern doctor might occasionally run across) and rickets (also a rare disease since acceptance of the value of cod liver oil used prophylactically). He was taught that all the essential elements are contained in a "balanced diet"—whatever that might be.

Anyone who reads the daily paper comes across that statement—about the "balanced diet"—every week or so from some doctor somewhere. It just isn't so, according to the report of the Department of Agriculture that was printed in the *Journal of the American Medical Association*—the doctors' bible!

To point out the errors in this concept would take a book. Indeed, it did take a book—a very excellent one that I have referred to already. I mean, of course, Dr. Roger J. Williams' *Nutrition Against Disease.*

A while ago I mentioned the desirability of a "nutritional checkup." In light of that, it is unfortunate that at present your doctor may well be the last person to whom you can go for advice on nutrition. This deficiency in the medical curriculum has been well described by Dr. J.E. Monagle, an M.D. who is Senior Consultant in Clinical Nutrition, Task Force on

Community Health, Health Programs Branch at Ottawa, Canada. In the *Canadian Doctor* for April 1973 Dr. Monagle said that although "the rudiments of nutrition [are] presented in basic sciences the practical utilization of that knowledge in clinical care is virtually ignored." He went on to describe a study at the Harvard School of Public Health in which the same tests on nutrition were given to graduating physicians, nurses, dietitians and high school students. "The physicians and nurses scored only marginally higher than the high school students." Dr. Monagle noted that the Commission on Nutrition Education and Training of the International Union of Nutritional Sciences has urged that nutrition be made a part of the clinical teaching in all medical schools.

During the last fifty years or so, the chemicalization of our foodstuffs has steadily diminished their nutritional content and added to them many chemicals whose functions are to prolong shelf life or to make the foods look more attractive or to make them taste better. (There are now between 2,500 and 3,000 synthetic flavors. Synthetic flavors and colors constitute about 80 percent of all food additives.)

In the United States Senate in April 1971 hearings were held on "Chemicals and the Future of Man." Here are the opening remarks of the Chairman, Senator Abraham Ribicoff:

> It is a common saying that we are what we eat. If this is true, then Americans are becoming a nation of processed, packaged, and preserved people. Last year, Americans bought more processed than fresh foods for the first time in our history. We spend more than 60 billion dollars for these convenience foods including such items as TV dinners, snack foods of all kinds, and frozen foods.
>
> With these foods we each consume every year more than four pounds of chemical preservatives, stabilizers, colorings, flavorings and other addi-

tives. And the amount of these artifificial substances is increasing every year. Their use has doubled in the past 15 years, from 400 million pounds to
more than 800 million pounds. Today, more than
3,000 chemicals are deliberately added to our foods.

These developments raise three basic questions:
(1) How much do we know about the hazards to
human health from these chemicals? (2) How much
assurance of chemical safety should we require?
and (3) What must the Federal Government do to
assure that the chemicals we absorb are safe?"

We know that a large number of these additives were
inadequately tested, and one large group of them have been
indicted as a primary, if not sole, cause of behavioral and
learning disabilities in children. These abnormalities have
increased steadily so that in California in the past ten to
twelve years, the incidence of hyperkinesia and learning difficulties has risen from 2 percent to an average of 20 to 25
percent and, in some cases, to 40 percent of an entire school
population. These figures are not related to the
socioeconomic status of the child or to his Intelligence Quo-
tient.

Dr. Ben Feingold of the Kaiser Foundation Hospital,
Permanente Group, told the section on Allergy of the convention of the American Medical Association in 1973 that he had
successfully treated, some hyperkinetic children with learning difficulties with the salicylate-free diet which eliminates
80 percent of the food additives, including artificial flavors
and colors. At the time the paper was presented he had
achieved "dramatic results" in fifteen to eighteen of twenty-
five such children merely by removing artificial flavoring and
coloring from their diets. When these substances were returned to their diets, these children returned to their former abnormal states. Since presentation of this paper Dr. Feingold

has treated more than fifty such children successfully and reports that other physicians have duplicated his results.

The eating habits of the average American school child, and probably even more significantly, the teenager, expose him to large quantities of these substances in hot dogs, cold cuts of meats, ice cream, soft drinks and ready-to-eat cereals. Artificial flavorings and colorings are contained, in fact, in 90 percent of processed foods.

And think of the possible effects of these chemicals on adults. They may well be the reason that sales of tranquilizers and sedatives have skyrocketed in the last few years or even for the fact that the number of "unpremeditated" murders and the number of suicides have risen.

What we must do, and it seems a hopeless task, is to educate the younger generation to avoid the dangers as much as possible and supplement their diets where needed. That means the addition of vitamins, minerals and amino acids. All this is well drawn up for you, as I have suggested, in Dr. Williams' book, *Nutrition Against Disease* and also in the various excellent books and scientific publications of Dr. Emmanuel Cheraskin.

The report of the Council on Foods and Nutrition which was published in the *Journal of the American Medical Association* in 1970 had a revealing title: it was known as the *Report on Malnutrition and Hunger in the United States*. It contains shocking revelations of the extent of both malnutrition and hunger, but although malnutrition is probably much more widespread than true hunger, it is "not as politically dramatic," to put it in the words used in the report itself. Yet malnutrition producing physiological impairments seems to be common. Conditions such as iron deficiency, growth impairment and obesity are widespread. Alarming amounts of goiter and rickets have been reported recently. This report states that "practically all deficiency disorders seen could have been prevented had patients and physicians had a proper understanding of nutrition and diet." Further, this report suggests that in spite of all this garnering of information, little if anything has been or is being done about the situation.

The report has had no real effect. We still read every day of how adequate the American diet is and how, therefore, supplementation is the idea of a few crackpots and a waste of money.

Is it possible, then, to get "an adequately balanced and nutritious diet" in the supermarket?

I think that it is a queer commentary on our society today that almost the only source of supply for wholesome and nutritious foodstuffs is the health food store, whose proprietors and customers have long been held up to derision by many medical journals and many medical men. The natural food and organic farming people have long been stigmatized as crackpots and food nuts. It may well be that the shoe is on the other foot and that they are the only rational and sensible purveyors of food.

How odd it is, too, that the essential vitamins and minerals needed to supplement our denuded diets are obtainable chiefly in these same health food stores! And how odd that although, as I have noted, there is now the beginning of a governmental effort to correct widespread malnutrition, the eating habits of the average child have long been condoned by the same government agencies who are also intent on preventing us from adding vitamin supplements to our woeful diets!

My older daughter Barbara is a speech therapist with preschool and elementary school patients. When I visited her last fall she showed me a seven-year-old child who was a real problem. He was hyperkinetic, had a very short attention span and exceedingly poor speech. She was helping him but not enough to suit her.

I suggested that she should start the boy on 800 IU of alpha tocopherol until I could send her an article I had, written by Dr. Alan Cott, a psychiatrist who had had success with such children using some of the megavitamins. The mother, a nurse, readily complied and by the time she had Dr. Cott's literature the child had become "perfectly normal," in the words of his mother and of the teachers in his school. He did not need further corrective therapy.

Barbara has since achieved the same result with a second child. The third mother to whom she suggested Vitamin E went to her own doctor for advice and was told that she would only be throwing her money away. So this child will need tranquilizers, sleeping pills and many hours of my daughter's professional help.

It is interesting that these profound changes occurred on Vitamin E alone. (Dr. Cott had not used Vitamin E in his megavitamin treatment.)

A newspaper report I saw not long ago quoted a prominent California lady as saying that people of her acquaintance who manage to look young and vital are often discovered to have been taking Vitamin E for years. Many athletes—including professional football players—are E users too.

Among athletes, in fact, the fame of Vitamin E seems even to have penetrated the Iron Curtain. I read in the 24 May 1972 issue of the *Medical Tribune* that young Soviet skiers and cyclists were given E during a study of E blood and urine levels at the Nutrition Institute of the Soviet Academy of Medical Science and the Central Institute of Physical Culture.

Commented the *Tribune* on the results: "We don't believe the Russians invented the electric light bulb—but are they among the first to demonstrate that increased physical activity raises requirements for Vitamin E?"

REFERENCES

1. *Journal of the American Medical Association* 213, 272, 1970.
2. *New England Journal of Medicine* 263, 379, 1960.

18

WHAT OF THE FUTURE?

THIS WAS THE TITLE of the last chapter in my last book! There I answered the question with a list of my hopes. Now, six years later, I can do better. For the future of alpha tocopherol therapy has, in the meantime, begun to take shape. The adoption of alpha tocopherol in the treatment of cardiovascular disease has been greatly accelerated since 1969, when my last book was published, in every state in the United States, in the British Isles, in Europe and in Australia and New Zealand.

Today, more cardiologists are realizing that they have virtually nothing to offer if they don't use alpha tocopherol and are at last investigating the claims for its use. Surgeons and family physicians are adopting alpha tocopherol treatment at a greater rate than the cardiologists. Now, even in articles blasting its use, they read admissions that it does work for humans in intermittent claudication, the anemias of premature infants and some other conditions. Obviously, since it works in these conditions, it is not an inert substance but is effective in treating very real pathological states in humans. As a result, they are motivated to investigate further.

The megavitamin way of using E—what I refer to as Big E, to contrast it with "little e," which is the use of E simply as a vitamin—is becoming more and more widespread. Big E is astonishingly and bewilderingly useful, and still more uses are being announced every year.

In addition to the steadily increasing number of doctors who find it useful, there is the size of the factories producing the concentrate and, especially, the millions of people using it daily. All these are a source of wonderment and joy to the Shute brothers who started it all. In Florida, where I now spend my winters, there is hardly a drug store in the state —and certainly no health food store—that doesn't have a most prominent display featuring Vitamin E. One drug store has a display showing two very tall basketball players advertising the house brand in 1,000 IU capsules. It is difficult to assess the accelerated rate of acceptance of alpha tocopherol therapy with great accuracy, since there are so many companies wholesaling Vitamin E capsules, most of them also selling directly to physicians. But it is safe to say that there has been more progress made in the last five years than in the previous twenty.

Invitations to present our work to professional groups are increasing in number. We have just no trouble at all in convincing the majority of those doctors who see our slides and learn of the literature that is available supporting our original claims. More and more doctors are hearing the message. As one young physician said when I lamented to him that his group was already using Big E and that I would prefer to address a group that was unfamiliar with it or skeptical,

"But we are all like amoebas. We have our tentacles out in our professional lives. Through us, other doctors have to listen to our successes with it."

So it is with our patients. They have persisted in getting well against their doctors' predictions. They have persisted in staying well and telling their friends how well Vitamin E works for them. Legions of them have solved their own problems after reading our papers or books. This we know from the literally thousands of letters we have received from some of them.

Many, many people have taken alpha tocopherol on their own responsibility. It works as well for them, of course, as it does for many patients treated with alpha tocopherol prescribed by a doctor, provided they have the right dosage for their pathological condition and have neither of the complaints in which Vitamin E can be dangerous, namely an elevated blood pressure or chronic rheumatic heart disease.

Here is nearly all of one typical—not unusual—letter from such a patient, one I have not seen:

> Dear Dr. Shute:
>
> May I introduce myself by saying that I have had a heart condition for nearly ten years, that I have read your book *Vitamin E for Ailing and Healthy Hearts*, and that I have been taking Vitamin E (1,200 IU) daily for the past seven months. To attempt to describe how I feel today almost defies description!
>
> I am 48 years old and suffered a myocardial infarction nearly ten years ago. After two months in the hospital, it was another six months before I was able to resume light activities. But this was not for long; a week later I experienced my second attack. In the years since then, I have had moments and times of considerable pain and distress. Next month,

November, will mark a year that I was forced to return to the States because of my heart condition. Upon arrival in the States, I was hospitalized for a month and a half.

Treatment, from the first time I was hospitalized and in the years since then, has consisted of daily medication; anticoagulant therapy, coronary dilators and treatment for high blood pressure.

Up until the time of my first heart condition, and in a very limited sense since then, my life had been quite active with a great part of it spent outdoors. Walking from 5 to 15 miles each day was common as there were no roads in the area that I was in. I had given up smoking and drinking (neither had ever been excessive) eight years before my first attack. Through necessity, because of scarcity, I had been on a relatively fat free diet—there were no dairy products available and even meat was a rare item. Rice was the main dish. My weight was not excessive—between slender and medium build. I had always enjoyed excellent health.

It was quite a change after my first and succeeding heart attacks. It became impossible to even attempt to walk briskly or to climb a hill. And while I was not aware of the high blood pressure condition before, there was no question about it afterwards and I had this problem since then. Needless to say, I was a bit discouraged when discharged from the hospital this last time and again looking forward to a future of daily medication and limited activity.

There has been an incredible change for the better in my heart and health since being introduced to your book and taking Vitamin E. I must truthfully admit that after finishing your book, I was still skeptical and had many unfounded reservations—that Vitamin E just wouldn't work in my particular case despite your claims and the many examples given. Fortunately for myself, my hopes were stronger than the doubts and I began with small and gradually increasing dosages of Vitamin E.

And now the part that defies description. I can actually run again—not as fast and as far as in times past—but maybe the years have something to do with that! Angina pains are a stranger to me now. My blood pressure over the past five months has averaged 130/83. The first day that I started with Vitamin E, I put the half empty bottles of [drugs prescribed for some heart patients] and those for high blood pressure and tension in my luggage. I have not used any of these drugs since then. Aside from having my blood pressure taken at intervals, I had one Prothrombin time taken a couple of weeks ago (control 12.8; patient, 12.3 seconds). I cannot begin to describe the change in my spirit, morale and physical well being. Those who "remember me before" are astounded at the rapidity and completeness of change for the better. Actually, I feel more like I did 15 or 20 years ago! . . .

Words are so meager and inadequate to express the extent of my gratitude to you but may I express it with a sincere and humble thank you. What words can a patient say to a doctor after a decade of living with an "ailing" and now . . . a healthy heart! Again, with my gratitude, prayers and best wishes,

Sincerely yours,
M.E.L.

It's hard to add anything to a letter like that. This patient has said a lot. I am very proud to have received such a letter and very happy that our work has made it possible for such a letter to be written.

I am also, personally, very proud to be included in symposia and scientific sessions with such intellectual and knowledgeable greats as Linus Pauling, Roger Williams, Emmanuel Cheraskin, Fred Klenner, Morgan Raiford, William Miller, Lyle Baker and the man with the encyclopedic knowledge of nutrition, Carlton Fredericks and many, many others also very knowledgeable. These men are changing the face of medicine.

I am grateful to the men who have formed what is now the International Academy of Preventive Medicine, since they have provided a platform for the meeting of minds and the dissemination of knowledge of the new medicine. Their membership, which now exceeds 500, includes people from most states.

I am inspired by the movement to form a similar group in Canada, which is just getting under way. Most of its personnel have attended meetings of the Academy in the United States either as speakers or listeners.

Gangrenous legs of diabetics are not all lopped off any more, and the use of Vitamin E ointment in burn cases as well as ulcers of all kinds, including bed sores, is rapidly being adopted by physicians across the country. With no particular fanfare or advertising of the ointment, sales are rapidly increasing. One convalescent and chronic-disease hospital in the East has been ordering the ointment not by the tube, not by the pound, but by the pail!

The heart transplant surgeon has virtually disappeared.

Indeed, I am exhilarated by the changes in the last six years. Yet in my happiness I am not disposed to be gentle with those who have opposed and criticized our work. My last book was gentle. This one is not! It is time that the opponents of Vitamin E therapy were deterred from further activity. It is time that the physician realizes that this treatment has come to stay. The time has come for the cardiologist to sit down and assess what he is doing for his patients, reconsider everything he has been taught, reconsider past recommendations and prescriptions, and consider the use of something which will help his patients' hearts—an antioxidant, a dissolver and preventer of intravascular clotting, and so a prophylaxis against man's killers.

I often wonder at the generosity of the American public. Each February the American Heart Association runs a campaign on radio and television and with volunteer door-to-door canvassers. These campaigns are run by professional fund raisers. In 1971 the American Heart Association allocated a record fifteen million dollars for research and in addition an estimated 8.5 million was allocated for research by state and community heart associations.

I am wondering when the generous American public is going to ask just what his millions of dollars contributed to this heart fund has netted. When will the average citizen become dissatisfied with the so-called basic research while he watches a type of heart disease unknown to Paul White at the time of his graduation in 1911 become the Number One killer of this generation?

The *Medical Post* for 12 January 1971 carried a report that should be interesting to my readers. It concerns the polyunsaturated fat diets so strongly recommended in the pamphlets put out by the American Heart Association. Some disturbing figures had turned up in "one of the largest and longest trials" of the antiatherosclerotic diet. Although those who had been on the diet had lower serum cholesterol and "few atherosclerotic episodes," they discovered that the group on the diet had "double the cancer mortality of controls matched for age, clinical condition and other parameters."

Since such a diet is deficient in Vitamin E, that article bears an obvious relationship to another that also appeared in the *Medical Post*, this one on 22 September 1970. Dr. Albert Barber, Professor of Zoology at the University of California at Los Angeles, is stated to have said that since Vitamin E is believed to protect unsaturated fats in the cells of the body, a deficiency may leave the cells "vulnerable to destruction by an environmental carcinogen." When the lipids in the cell membrane are destroyed by oxidation, "the membrane breaks up and the cell loses a growth-control factor." Dr. Barber thinks that if his idea is borne out, E could be useful in preventing cancer.

Some work along somewhat similar lines was announced in the *Montreal Star* for 30 July 1973. According to the *Star*, two scientists at Sir George Williams University, Montreal, have been following a lead provided fifty years ago by the German physiologist Otto Warburg, who worked on the theory that lack of oxygen in a cell might lead to the formation of tumors. Professor Adolph E. Smith of Sir George Williams University was quoted as saying, "If a cell doesn't get enough oxygen it is possible it may resort to a different way of life."

It is interesting to note that the two scientists mentioned immediately above had published in a Swiss scientific magazine. Notice how often American and Canadian scientists publish their work in the English medical magazine *The Lancet*. Note also that the numerous papers mentioned here as presented to the various medical conventions, even the annual and specialist groups of the American Medical Association and the American Heart Association, seldom see the light of day in the medical journals put out by the American Medical Association or the American Heart Association. Perhaps this is why the American Medical Association is faced with declining membership and revenues and has had to make a series of belt-tightening moves aimed at saving over one million dollars per year. Nine councils and committees have been dropped at a saving of $840,000. Subscriptions to some of its magazines are no longer free. A variety of other moves have been undertaken to save funds and streamline the Association. It has just been announced by Dr. Philip L. White, chairman, that the A.M.A. Council on Foods and Nutrition has been placed on "inactive status" because of budget costs.

Returning to the consideration of cancer and Vitamin E, it is worth reporting that all those concerned in my practice have remarked many times in the last few years that very, very few of our patients develop cancer. Vitamin E is certainly not the only factor, since the occasional patient does develop cancer, but again very, very few do. This is all the more remarkable considering the older age group into which most of our patients fall.

We have steered clear of any claim concerning cancer, and I mention it now only because of the three items above.

As I come to the end of this book, a final thought strikes me. Throughout the entire eighteen chapters I have never mentioned sex. And yet for years it was widely believed by people who knew very little about Vitamin E that it was "the sex vitamin." This misconception arose, apparently, from the very real fact that it did help childless couples to have families. But no one familiar with Big E has ever claimed that it has aphrodisiac powers, least of all our group. The one book on the subject produces no evidence whatsoever. The author's thesis is that people on Vitamin E often feel much better and that in better health, one may be a better performer! Let me add to that one observation directed at heart patients. They should be taking appropriate quantities of E because it's a lot sexier to be ALIVE!

APPENDIX A

VITAMIN E
AS A THERAPEUTIC AGENT
IN DERMATOLOGY

Reprinted from *Current News in Dermatology* for March, 1973 by courtesy of Arthur G. Schoch, M.D., Editor.

Samuel Ayres, Jr. of Los Angeles, wrote us on request on "Vitamin E as a Therapeutic Agent in Dermatology." We quote his letter in its entirety:

Dr. Richard Mihan and I became interested in Vitamin E when Milton Stout presented before the Los Angeles Dermatological Society in 1950, a woman with pseudoxanthoma elasticum whose cutaneous and visual impairment were restored to near normal following administration of Vitamin E for a period of 1 year (*Arch. Derm.* 60:310, 1951).

This astounding therapeutic accomplishment in a hitherto untreatable disease led us to carry out a continuing clinical investigation among our private office patients with some highly gratifying results. We were able to confirm Stout's results in 1 case of pseudoxanthoma elasticum.

Another disease involving elastic tissues, epidermolysis bullosa, has also responded to large doses of Vitamin E. We have successfully treated 2 patients with the simplex type, confirming a previous report by H.D. Wilson (*Can. Med. Assoc. J.* 901:1315, 1964). Our findings have in turn been confirmed by Sehgal et al. (*Dermatologica*, 144:27, 1927), and by John Knox at the December 1972 convention of the American Academy of Dermatology, where he showed slides illustrating the clinical and histological response to Vitamin E in 3 cases of epidermolysis bullosa dystrophica.

We have had gratifying results with Vitamin E in a limited number of cases of other recalcitrant dermatoses of obscure etiology, including Raynaud's phenomenon with gangrene, scleroderma, calcinosis cutis (*Cutis*, 11:54, 1973), Darier's disease (in combination with Vitamin A), several types of cutaneous vasculitis, subcorneal pustular dermatosis, benign chronic familial pemphigus, and some cases of chronic ulcers, discoid lupus erythematosus and granuloma annulare.

As a beneficial side-effect it was noted that Vitamin E gave prompt relief to severe nocturnal leg cramps, which in turn led to a hobby of successfully treating various types of muscle spasms, including not only nocturnal leg cramps, but also intermittent claudication, exercise cramps, restless legs syndrome, etc., when the patient's history revealed their presence (*Calif. Med.* 111: 87-91, 1969 and *JAMA* 219:216-217, 1972).

Vitamin E has several important functions including its antitoxidant effect in protecting unstable lipoprotein membranes of cells and intracellular organelles from peroxidative destruction, while at the same time promoting oxygen utilization in normal metabolic processes (*Geriatrics* 23:97, 1968 and *Vitamins and Hormones* 20:541, 1954). It also has vital relationships with certain enzymes, trace minerals such as selenium, with other vitamins.

The question as to whether or not a certain individual is receiving the so-called minimum daily requirement of Vitamin E is irrelevant. Adequate intake is only one aspect. Absorption and utilization are equally important and various factors of congenital or acquired origin may result in defective utilization of Vitamin E, which in turn may lead to a wide spectrum of pathological changes. We would emphasize, therefore, that we have employed Vitamin E not as a vitamin supplement, but as a potent therapeutic agent. In the conditions mentioned above, we have usually prescribed Vitamin E as d-alpha- tocopheryl acetate in doses from 400 IU to 800 IU daily, and in some cases up to 1600 or 2000 IU daily. We have encountered no untoward side-effects. Patients with severe hypertension, serious cardiac impairment, or diabetics on insulin should be started on much smaller doses such as 100 IU daily, which can be gradually increased over a period of weeks or several months. Simultaneous administration of iron inactivates Vitamin E. Vitamin E topically in the form of drops or a cream is also useful.

We have had no experience with Vitamin E in progeria, but theoretically it should prove effective, if begun early in life. Hans Selye was able to induce a progeria-like syndrome in rats by feeding Vitamin D_2 and he was able to block it simultaneously by administering Vitamin E (*Am. Report to Distillation Products Industries* 6:7, 1963).

The rarity of some of the dermatoses under consideration precludes the use of double blind controlled studies, but we hope that other dermatologists will try this simple, innocuous therapeutic agent in some of these recalcitrant dermatoses."

APPENDIX B

AN EXCERPT FROM AN ARTICLE BY LADY PHILLIS CILENTO

●

(Excerpted from an article which appeared in *Woman's Day*, an Australian weekly magazine, for 12 November 1973.)

FACTS I FOUND

At the beginning of this series I said that my aim was to discover the truth about Vitamin E.

There is no question in my mind but that I have done this. From what I have seen and learnt overseas, coupled with my own experience and that of doctors like Reid Tweedie in Malaysia, Dr. R.T. of London, Mr. Lambert of Dublin, Dr. Beckmann of Germany and of Drs. Evan and Wilfrid Shute, I am convinced that the claims made for alpha-tocopherol are fully justified.

With my own eyes I have seen pictures proving the almost miraculous effects of the vitamin on severe burns.

I have seen bent and stiffened fingers (Dupuytren's contracture) extend and become almost normal in five weeks of treatment with alpha-tocopherol.

I have seen ulcers, eczema, gangrene disappear; I have seen wounds that had failed to respond to skin grafting healed with scarcely a scar, and I have seen new (collateral) circulation forming under the influence of alpha-tocopherol in animals, in which occlusion of a blood vessel has been artificially induced.

I have seen angina cases lose their pain and circulation in the legs and feet restored, and I have seen coronary sufferers regain their vigor, their interest in life and their capacity for work.

At the end of this article I shall set out exactly the way Vitamin E has been shown to work in the body. However, firstly, I want to emphasize that Vitamin E is only *one* vitamin, and since all vitamins interact and balance one another, it works better in company with other vitamins such as A,B, and C.

Also, as many of the diseases which Vitamin E benefits are caused by a number of factors, better results are obtained when alpha-tocopherol forms part of a general regimen of treatment. The other factors should not be neglected.

For example, in preventing coronary thrombosis or in rehabilitating a damaged heart, Vitamin E. though an essential factor, is more effective when aided by suitable exercise, balanced diet, no smoking, certain drugs and a tranquil mind, than when working alone.

●

Whenever I hear people ridiculing the claims of the Shutes, calling them "cranks" and refusing to consider the possibility that Vitamin E may have a saving function in cardiovascular disease, I look again at the list of deaths from heart disease in Australia.

Between 1950 and 1971 deaths from heart disease have climbed inexorably from 37,849 or 48.41 per cent of all deaths to 60,612 or 54.77 per cent of all deaths, despite the present methods being used and the millions of dollars being spent on research, which does *NOT* include Vitamin E.

The Heart Foundation here in Australia has so far refused even to consider investigating the value of Vitamin E in cardiovascular disease or of making trials of its use.

I am reminded of the many other occasions when life-saving innovations were delayed for years by the irrational conservatism of the medical Establishment:

How Lind was scoffed and attacked by his superiors and colleagues for 47 years after his discovery of the saving qualities of lemon juice for scurvy.

How it took 14 years and the necessities of war before the properties of penicillin were conceded and utilized.

How I, myself, was ridiculed and dismissed as a crank by a distinguished medical teacher when in 1919 I advocated Vitamin D for cases of severe rickets. I was laughed at even though, at that time, the vitamin was curing starving babies in war-torn Vienna of this deforming disease.

And I am reminded of great men like Pasteur and his work on anthrax, Jenner and smallpox, Semmelweiss and childbed fever.

To the list of such men who fought the good fight against conservatism and uninformed opinion, history must now add Evan and Wilfrid Shute.

For I have seen what Vitamin E can do, and I am certain that it is destined to play as great a role in the reduction of coronary heart disease as Vitamin C has done in saving thousands of sailors from death by scurvy over the past 200 years.

Once Vitamin E jumps the barriers of prejudice, it may

well be instrumental in saving the lives and sparing the suffering of many thousands of Australians who will otherwise die.

HOW VITAMIN E WORKS IN THE BODY

1. First and foremost it *reduces the need of the tissue cells for oxygen*, by preventing their destruction by over-oxidation with the formation of harmful products. Where the blood supply which carries oxygen to every cell is lessened, Vitamin E conserves that oxygen, and so the life and usefulness of the cells are preserved.

2. It *prevents clotting* in blood vessels (thrombosis) but does not prevent normal clotting after an injury.

3. It also *melts fresh clots* and dissolves some old ones.

4. It *opens up new channels* of blood supply when others are blocked and so improves circulation to a "half dead" area—such as in coronary occlusion.

5. It *dilates the smallest blood vessels*, the capillaries, which actually bring the blood in contact with the tissues, and delivers oxygen and nourishment where it is needed most. This aids the healing of burns and ulcers.

6. It *prevents the formation of hard scar tissue*, softens old scars, prevents their contraction and so avoids deformities after burns and injuries.

7. It increases and sets free *blood platelets* when they are needed for normal clotting in wounds.

8. It improves the action of *insulin in diabetes* and prevents many complications of this disease.

9. It regulates the use of *proteins and fats* in the body.

10. It *stimulates the flow of urine* and the action of kidneys and so reduces retention of fluid in the tissues (edema).

11. It preserves the *walls of the red-blood cells* and prevents their destruction, especially when almost pure oxygen is breathed—as with premature babies in humidicribs and astronauts in space capsules.

12. It increases the *power and activity of muscle cells*—heart muscle as well as ordinary muscles.

13. In the *veterinary field* Vitamin E improves the stamina and speed of racing dogs and horses, and improves the fertility of stud animals.

14. It improves the number and activity of the *male sperm cells* in the semen.

15. It normalizes the *activity of the ovaries in women*, improving the periods and preventing many menopausal symptoms such as excessive bleeding, dryness and irritation of the genital organs.

16. It maintains the health and normal blood supply to the unborn baby in the early weeks of its life in the womb and *prevents many types of miscarriages*. This was first observed in the rat and other animals, but was later found to be equally valuable for the foetus (early unborn baby).

17. Vitamin E assists the absorption and action of Vitamin A and other vitamins in the body.

APPENDIX C

IS COMMERCIALISM CONTROLLING THE CONTROVERSY OVER CHOLESTEROL?

This is an abstract of an article by E.R. Pinkney which appeared in *Medical Counterpoint* for May 1971. The abstract appeared in *The Summary*, a publication of the Shute Foundation for Medical Research, London, Ontario, Canada. It is reprinted here with the permission of the Foundation.

There is still no good clinical evidence that a diet-lowered serum cholesterol in any way prevents or modifies heart attacks or heart disease.

And yet for over twelve years a large number of physicians have attempted to control their patients' serum cholesterol.

The World Heath Organization reports an *increase* in morbidity and mortality from atherosclerotic heart disease. By contrast, in Japan, the consumption of dairy products, eggs and saturated fats has increased greatly since 1955. But that country had a 14 percent decrease in heart deaths for the same period.

There has been practically no change in the cholesterol consumed over the past 60 years. But in the same era the heart attack rate has climbed rapidly.

Those who believe in the relationship of serum cholesterol to coronary heart disease find that no test proved more helpful than an accurate total serum cholesterol. The measurement of serum cholesterol has become the principal indicator of the health of one's heart and blood vessels to both public and the medical profession alike.

Any stress, small or great, can alter the level of serum cholesterol.

Advertising P.U.F.A.* as helpful for hearts is permitted—even in reputable medical journals, although there is not a bit of proof to back such claims. Simultaneously the Food and Drug Administration requires a most specific disclaimer of any positive relationship between the lowering of cholesterol and the prevention of coronary heart disease. Since 1959 the F.D.A. has threatened to prosecute any manufacturer who relates polyunsaturates to the prevention of heart disease but no action has been taken to this moment. The ads still appear.

There is ample evidence that heating polyunsaturates tend to resaturate (or polymerize) the product and so defeats the very purpose for which polyunsaturates are promoted. Resaturation of polyunsaturates by heating occurs in family cooking. The degree of saturation becomes even worse if the fat or oil is reused, as is common household practice.

Heating an unsaturated oil (especially corn oil) to 200° for 15 minutes (far less than normal cooking temperatures and time) actually enhances atherosclerosis in animals.

In Kummerow's study all his animals on a diet containing

*Polyunsaturated fatty acids. [Ed.]

heated corn oil developed tumors, and only one of 96 survived the 40-month experimental period. None of the animals fed only fresh corn oil developed tumors; all survived.

Men on a high P.U.F.A. diet showed a 65 percent greater incidence of cancer than controls on a standard diet. The *J.A.M.A.* reporting this finding also noted that those on the high P.U.F.A. diet also had 70 fatal atherosclerotic accidents as compared to only 48 such deaths in the controls; a similar ratio was found for myocardial and cerebral infarcts.

Polyunsaturates may be a primary source of the radicals inside the cell that cause aging.

The serum cholesterol level falls only three mgm for each 100 mgm of cholesterol taken out of the diet.

After 20 years of low fat diets and the spending of several hundred million dollars, there is still no convincing evidence for this idea that these fats matter.

Yet even the eminent National Heart and Lung Institute has lately published a set of guidelines for physicians. This recommends that certain individuals with an elevated serum cholesterol should use polyunsaturates.

One cannot show that, subsequent to reduction of patient's serum cholesterol values, the cholesterol itself actually leaves the body.

AUTHOR'S ADDENDUM

SINCE THE COMPLETION of the majority of the work on this book, new statistics have become available which shed a somewhat different—and very interesting—light on death from heart disease in the American population.

Although the total number of deaths per hundred thousand from heart disease has risen during the past couple of decades, it appears that deaths from heart disease and some other causes have been declining when measured on an age-adjusted basis—a statistical approach which takes into account the fact that the average age is increasing.

Then, on January 24, 1975, at an American Heart Association Seminar, Dr. Jeremiah Stamler announced that the heart attack rate among American men had started a downward trend for the first time.

Anyone who has read all the way through this book,

should feel no surprise. The whole point of the book is the contrast between the ineffectiveness of orthodox treatment and prevention of cardiovascular disease, and the effective treatment and prevention of cardiovascular disease with adequate Vitamin E therapy. Thirty million Americans taking Vitamin E had to produce such a reduction, and the 10,000 lives saved in 1974 has to be just about that anticipated after six years of prophylactic E in such a large section of the population.

If there is any other explanation, it has not been suggested so far. The last paragraph in my book *Vitamin E for Ailing and Healthy Hearts* reads as follows:

"My father saw few cases of coronary occlusion and few diabetics. I have seen thousands. There was no coronary thrombosis in 1900. There need be none in the year 1980. It's up to you now."

Now, six years later, it seems that such a hope just could be within our grasp.

Wilfrid E. Shute, B.A., M.D.
Lake Worth, Florida
February 22, 1975

INDEX